CW00347022

Herbal Remedies
For Beginners

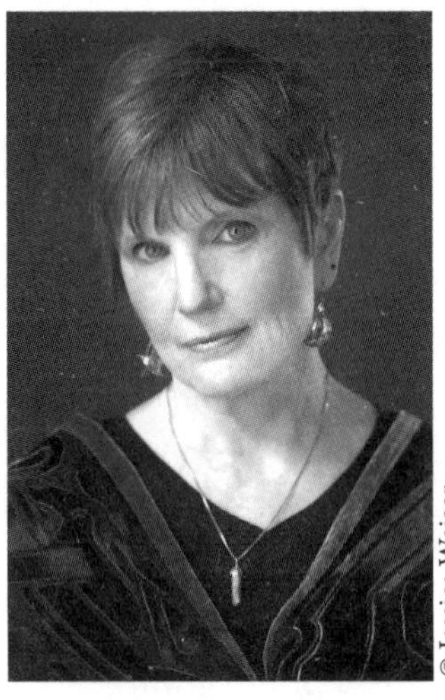

© Jessica Weiser

About the Author

Sandra Kynes is a Reiki practitioner and a member of the Bards, Ovates & Druids. She likes to develop creative ways to explore the world and integrate them into her spiritual path, which serves as the basis for her books. Sandra has lived in New York City, Europe, England, and now coastal New England. She loves connecting with nature through gardening, hiking, bird watching, and ocean kayaking. Visit her website at www.kynes.net.

Herbal Remedies

For Beginners

Natural Ways to Treat Ailments

Sandra Kynes

Llewellyn Publications
Woodbury, Minnesota

First Edition
First Printing, 2020

Cover design by Shannon McKuhen

Library of Congress Cataloging-in-Publication Data (Pending)
978-0-7387-6191-6

Llewellyn Publications
A Division of Llewellyn Worldwide Ltd.
2143 Wooddale Drive
Woodbury, MN 55125-2989
www.llewellyn.com

Printed in the United States of America

Other Books by Sandra Kynes

Magical Symbols and Alphabets (2020)

365 Days of Crystal Magic (2018)

Crystal Magic (2017)

Plant Magic (2017)

Bird Magic (2016)

The Herb Gardener's Essential Guide (2016)

Star Magic (2015)

Llewellyn's Complete Book of Correspondences (2013)

Mixing Essential Oils for Magic (2013)

Change at Hand (2009)

Sea Magic (2008)

Your Altar (2007)

Whispers from the Woods (2006)

A Year of Ritual (2004)

Gemstone Feng Shui (2002)

contents

introduction

There are many reasons to use herbal remedies. Increasingly, one of the most important is that they help us avoid putting more unnecessary chemicals into and onto our bodies. Over-the-counter remedies often contain ingredients such as sorbitol, parabens, and a range of other binders, fillers, and preservatives that can cause negative side effects. In contrast, we know exactly what is in the remedies we make. Plus, herbs offer a holistic way to deal with common health issues.

Although chemicals were used extensively in manufacturing medicines and other products during the twentieth century, the rise of the ecology movement raised awareness about the use of them. Shifting attitudes ushered in an interest in and revival of herbal medicine and other natural healing methods and disciplines. As more of these "alternatives" continue to make their way into mainstream acceptance, we are finding that a mix of traditional herbal and conventional medicine can give us the best of both worlds. Another advantage of herbal remedies is that unlike conventional medicine, which treats symptoms, herbs also aid in establishing wellness and support good health. That said, we must keep safety in mind because herbs are powerful and must be used properly.

I grew up in a household where the first line of defense against illness and the first aid rendered after injury came from the kitchen or my grandmother's garden. While commercial products eventually made their way into the family medicine cabinet (*new* and *convenient* were the buzzwords of the early 1960s), my mother often went back to the remedies she knew as a child. Because of that, I became familiar with them, too. Well, I knew that they looked and smelled different from the stuff that came from the store.

When I went off to college in New York City, I did what most young people do and used the same store-bought products that everyone else used. I drifted away from homemade remedies. I was clueless about how to make them, anyway. Years later, childhood memories and the desire to move away from chemical-based products piqued my interest in herbal medicine. At the time, I was living overseas in the pre-Internet era when communications were much slower and international phone calls were very expensive. So, I did what you are doing now—I read books.

Although the books I bought were helpful, I found myself wishing for one that combined the best of all of them. The most important component, of course, is being able to look up an ailment to find which herbs and application methods to use. However, because I didn't have a wide range of herbs on hand, I thought it would be nice to be able to look up an herb to see what ailments it can be used to treat. I also appreciated books that had a basic section on how to make the various remedies so I didn't have to skim through all the pages looking for instructions for a particular one. Last but not least, I wanted a book that was more than just recipes, one that would give me a better understanding of common ailments and what types of treatments and remedies were effective. I wanted holistic information.

My goal for this project has been to put together a "best of" book that provides an introduction and foundation for making remedies and working with herbs, but also serves as a comprehensive reference for years to come. To that end, Chapter 1 provides the lowdown on botanical names, information on where to buy herbs if you don't grow your own, an overview on dosages, what equipment is needed, and much more to get you started. Chapters 2 and 3 provide information on how to make and use various types of remedies from a simple tea to a beeswax ointment. Although recipes are given throughout the book, it is important to read the full descriptions provided in these chapters. They also serve as a go-to reference as you try new remedies and incorporate new herbs into your repertoire.

Focusing on first aid, Chapter 4 contains remedies that you can whip up quickly and others you may want to make ahead of time to have on hand. Chapters 6 through 12 focus on individual systems or parts of the body and the remedies that can be used to deal with common ailments.

Chapters 13 and 14 contain brief profiles of the herbs mentioned throughout this book. Each profile includes the plant's description, scientific name, precautions and contraindications, and medicinal uses so you can get the most from the herbs you have on hand. In addition to herbs, Chapter

14 contains details on several commonly used base ingredients, such as cocoa butter, beeswax, aloe vera gel, and others. Because these ingredients also have some healing properties, this information can help you plan and make remedies that are best for you.

Appendix A provides a convenient alphabetical listing of all the ailments covered in this book. It also serves as a quick reference for the herbs and other ingredients that can be used for each ailment. Appendix B contains measurement equivalents to help you determine the easiest way to measure ingredients for your preparations.

Even if you are already working with herbs, this book will serve as a convenient reference on herbal remedies to support healing and good health for you and your family.

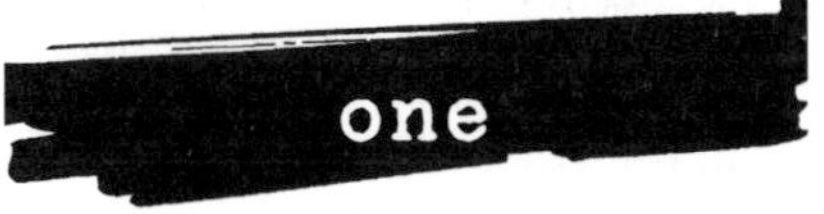

Getting Started

Making herbal remedies is an empowering and fun experience. While it may seem as though there is so much to learn when you are just getting started, don't feel daunted; you don't need to know everything immediately. Working with herbs is a journey, not a destination. You can start with one of your favorite herbs and learn its medicinal uses. Or, you can start with an ailment and learn which herbs can be used to treat it and sometimes keep it from recurring. As you go along, you will learn what you need to know for you and your family because you will be able to tailor remedies to your specific needs and preferences.

While a number of recipes in this book include more than one herb, you do not need a long list of ingredients to make an effective remedy. In fact, for centuries herbalists prepared medicines known as simples, remedies made with only one herb. Working with one herb is a good way to get to know it and understand how it works for you. The recipes in this book are suggestions, and for most of them, you can substitute any of the other herbs listed for an ailment.

Making our own remedies is also like a little adventure where we get to experiment and work with ingredients that we may not have used before. That is one reason why I recommend making remedies in small amounts. Another reason is to have fresh ones on hand.

The Importance of Scientific Names

While the common names of plants are easy to remember, they can be a source of confusion because a plant may be known by multiple names or two plants can share a common name. For example, there are several types of lavender, which makes it important to purchase the right one. For the purposes described in this book, English lavender (*Lavandula angustifolia*, syn. *L. officinalis*) is the one to buy. Spanish lavender (*L. stoechas*) is a stimulating herb and has the opposite effect of English lavender. Spanish lavender is also called French lavender.

Genus and species are part of a complex naming structure devised by Swedish naturalist Carl Linnaeus (1707–1778) whose work became the foundation for the International Code of Botanical Nomenclature. Over time, as new knowledge about plants emerged, their names were changed to reflect the new data or correct mistakes.

This is one reason why we find synonyms in botanical names as noted above with English lavender. The antiquated names are not completely dropped because they aid in identification. For example, the botanical names for German chamomile are noted as *Matricaria recutita*, syn. *M. chamomilla*, and black cohosh as *Actaea racemosa*, syn. *Cimicifuga racemosa*. Other reasons for the use of synonyms are scientific disagreement and sometimes stubbornness.

The names are in Latin because during Linnaeus's time it was a common language for people engaged in scientific research. The first word in a botanical name is the plant's genus, which is often a proper noun and always capitalized. Because aloe vera is also the plant's common name, the word *aloe* is only capitalized when referring to the botanical name.

The second word, the species name, is an adjective that usually provides something descriptive about the plant. For example, the genus for coriander, *Coriandrum*, is the Latin name for the plant, which was derived from the Greek *koriannon*. The species name, *sativum*, means "cultivated" as opposed to a plant that is gathered from the wild.[1]

Often used as species names, the terms *officinalis* and *officinale* indicate that an herb was an official medicinal plant of apothecaries and physicians when it was named. Examples include ginger, *Zingiber officinale*, and lemon balm, *Melissa officinalis*.[2] In the botanical names for thyme and oregano (*Thymus vulgaris* and *Origanum vulgare*) the terms *vulgare* and *vulgaris* do not refer to coarse manners but indicate that it is a common species of plant.[3]

You may also see the letter *X* in a name, which indicates that the plant is a hybrid, a cross between two plants. For example, peppermint, *Mentha x piperita*, is a naturally occurring hybrid between spearmint (*M. spicata*) and water mint (*M. aquatica*). A letter or abbreviation sometimes follows

1. Cumo, *Encyclopedia of Cultivated Plants*, 436.

2. Madison, *The Illustrated Encyclopedia of Fruits*, 270.

3. Neal, *Gardener's Latin*, 133.

a botanical name and identifies the person who named the plant. For example, "F. Meull" is the abbreviation for Ferdinand von Mueller (1825–1896), a German-Australian botanist. The letter *L* at the end of a botanical name means that Linnaeus himself bestowed the name.

While it is not necessary to memorize botanical names, it is helpful to jot them down so you can have them handy when shopping for herbs. As mentioned, getting the correct one is important because even similar herbs can have different properties and, more importantly, different precautions and contraindications.

General Precautions

Although I like to encourage people to explore, have fun, and reap the benefits of herbs without feeling intimidated by not being an expert, working with herbs must be done with knowledge and common sense. Although they are natural alternatives to synthetic, chemical-based treatments, herbs must be used with safety in mind. They are powerful healers that can be harmful when not used properly. For each herb you use, it is important to read the precautions and contraindications in the profiles provided in Chapters 13 and 14 and any safety guidelines provided by a vendor. Depending on the ailment you are treating, you may want to speak with your doctor before using herbs, especially if you are taking any type of medication.

When you use an herbal remedy internally for the first time, start with a small amount to make sure you do not have an adverse reaction. If you have any sign of nausea, diarrhea, stomach upset, or headache, discontinue it immediately. Herbal remedies are generally not recommended for internal use by children under two years of age, and when given to an older child they should be diluted—never a full-strength adult dosage. Women who are pregnant or nursing must be sure to follow precautions carefully and are advised to first consult their physician or specialist. Anyone taking a prescription medication should consult their doctor before using herbs as they can interact with some drugs.

It is important to work with your doctor when ailments are prolonged or if they escalate. Luckily, more physicians are open to "alternative" treatments and working with their patients rather than dictating to them.

Sources for Herbs

Growing our own herbs is the best way to ensure top quality and there are plenty of books on the subject, including my own *The Herb Gardener's Essential Guide*. If having a garden or even growing them on a windowsill is not possible or convenient, there are alternatives such as buying dried herbs or fresh ones that you can dry yourself. Dried herbs are available at supermarkets, health food stores, specialty tea shops, and online.

Reading labels is most important. First, check the botanical name to be sure you are getting the right one. Look for herbs that are organic and non-GMO (genetically modified organism). Organic products should be certified and have a USDA label, which means they were grown and handled according to standards established by the United States Department of Agriculture. These standards also require growers to protect natural resources, promote ecological balance, and conserve biodiversity.

You may encounter some labels that include notations such as *grown without chemicals or pesticides*, which does not mean the product is organic or that the environmental guidelines were followed. The term *natural* is completely meaningless. Herbs come from nature; therefore, they are natural.

Before buying online, check around. Use social media to ask for other people's experiences with a vendor. Contact the vendor if you have questions; reputable sellers will answer customers' inquiries. In addition to botanical names, a seller should provide information on which products are USDA-certified organic and where the plants are grown.

While it may be tempting to buy in bulk for better pricing, keep in mind that herbs lose taste and potency over time. Buy small amounts when trying herbs for the first time to make sure you like them and that they work for you. On the other hand, if you use certain herbs frequently, buying in bulk may be better. Over time, you will be able to gauge how much to buy.

Farmers markets are an excellent source for fresh herbs. Take time to speak with vendors because they are often the people who grew the plants. Market vendors are usually delighted to share their knowledge and are often a good source of information.

Drying Herbs

While fresh herbs are wonderful to work with, most of us do not live in areas that allow us to grow them outdoors or buy them fresh at farmers markets all year round. The solution is to dry your own. Air-drying herbs by hanging them in bunches is an easy way to preserve them.

Air-drying works best in a dark or semi-dark location with low humidity, good airflow, and a steady, warm temperature. It is important to bundle the same type of herb together rather than mixing them because different types of plants dry at different rates. Basil, lemon balm, and the mints have high moisture contents and dry more slowly than some others such as sage, rosemary, and thyme.

Usually, up to ten stems can be tied into a bundle. Herbs that take longer to dry should be tied into smaller bundles of about five or fewer. Attach several bunches upside down to a wire coat hanger with enough space between them to allow air to circulate freely around the herbs. A wooden laundry rack can be placed wherever the conditions are right, and it can hold a number of herb-ladened coat hangers. If you don't have a lot of herbs to dry, the bunches can be attached directly to the laundry rack.

Whichever way you hang them, make sure the bunches are not touching each other and that they are not against a wall or other structure that would inhibit airflow. If you are concerned about dust, tie a piece of cheesecloth around each bundle of herbs or drape it over the whole laundry rack, if you are using one. Check the bundles every day and take them down as soon as they are dry; they should feel slightly brittle.

If you live in a small apartment or just don't have the space for hanging them, using the oven is a quicker way to dry herbs. Place paper towels on a cookie sheet, and then spread out the herbs in one even layer. Set the oven at the lowest temperature and leave the herbs in for two to four hours. Keep the oven door slightly ajar to allow air movement and to keep the herbs from baking. Check them every hour and turn them over once or twice for uniform drying. When they are crisp, remove them from the oven. Prolonged exposure to heat can cause them to lose flavor and potency. Allow the herbs to cool completely before storing.

Whichever method you use, once the herbs are dry, strip the leaves and/or flowers from the stems and store them in an airtight container immediately, otherwise they will start to deteriorate. Use glass jars with tight-fitting lids and avoid metal containers as they can taint the herbs. Store the jars in a cool place away from direct sunlight. Dried herbs can keep for up to a year or a little longer. If you notice a mist or moisture inside a jar, take the herbs out and dry them a bit more. Make sure the jar is dry before storing them again.

If you are drying roots, cut them into small pieces first. Place a layer of paper towels on a cookie sheet and spread out the root pieces in one layer. Set the oven at the lowest temperature for three to four hours. Leave the door ajar to allow air circulation and to keep the roots from baking. Turn them for uniform drying. Transfer the roots to a screen and place it in a warm room to complete the drying process, which can take up to two weeks.

Freezing is another method for preserving herbs. It works especially well for basil, dill, fennel, lemongrass, the mints, parsley, and thyme. Some herbs such as basil may lose color and texture, but they retain their flavor and potency. To prepare herbs for freezing, lay them out in a single layer on a baking sheet, and then place it in the freezer. Once the herbs are frozen, store them in containers. Herbs can be frozen whole, or they can be chopped. When making remedies with frozen herbs, thaw and drain them first to reduce their water content.

Equipment for Making Remedies

Chances are you already have most of what you need for making remedies because fancy equipment is not necessary. When preparing remedies, use stainless-steel sieves and glass, enamel, or stainless-steel pots and pans. Avoid aluminum because the herbs can absorb chemicals from the metal and potentially become toxic. Before pouring boiling water or anything hot into a container, especially if it is glass, warm it with hot tap water to prevent it from cracking or shattering. Pre-warming a cup or jar helps keep an infusion or tea warm while it steeps.

Be sure all utensils and containers for making and storing remedies are clean and dry. Basic equipment for making herbal remedies includes the following:

- Various-size saucepans
- Stockpot for when a large amount of an infusion is needed
- Double boiler for hot oil infusions
- Measuring cups and spoons
- Glass or ceramic bowls
- Various-size glass jars with tight-fitting lids
- Mortar and pestle for crushing seeds
- Fine-mesh sieves, a small one for tea and a larger one for infusions and decoctions

- Muslin cloth or bags (cheesecloth is too loosely woven for herbs)
- Tea filter bags for small poultices
- Small bottles with dropper tops for tinctures
- Pen and paper, computer, or cell phone for taking notes
- Small adhesive labels or masking tape

Not all the equipment is needed at once; you can acquire what you need as you go along or use what you have on hand. For example, instead of using a glass jar for steeping infusions, a teapot or French press can be used.

A double boiler is a set of saucepans that fit together. The larger bottom pan is used to boil water to create steam to warm the smaller upper pan. The upper saucepan has a lid. Because the heat is indirect, food and remedies do not burn. Also known by the French term *bain marie*, a double boiler is the preferred method for cooking delicate sauces, custards, crème brûlée, and chocolate. In place of a double boiler, a large stainless-steel mixing bowl can be placed over a large saucepan of water. You will need a lid to cover the bowl. The bottom of the bowl should not touch the water in the pan because the contents may overheat. Use oven mitts to lift the bowl from the saucepan.

The final step after making an herbal remedy is to label it. There are many sizes of adhesive labels on the market, but in a pinch, a piece of masking tape will do. Label your remedy with the date, the herbs, and any other ingredients used to make it.

Dosages

One of the wonderful things about herbal remedies is that we can tailor them to our specific needs; however, in the beginning it may seem a little daunting to figure out how much to use. When using an herb for the first time, go minimal to determine the amount that is effective for you. Topical applications are relatively easy to gauge the herb's effectiveness. The internal use of teas, infusions, decoctions, syrups, and tinctures are not as straightforward. The following general guidelines are based on an average adult weighing 150 pounds. You will need to adjust accordingly:

- Tea, infusion, decoction—up to 3 or 4 cups a day
- Syrup—up to 6 or 8 teaspoons a day
- Tincture—up to 2 or 4 teaspoons a day

Another thing to consider is whether the ailment is acute (rapid onset and lasting for a short period) or chronic (persistent and of long duration). For acute problems, take dosages in smaller amounts more frequently. For example, if the dosage is 3 cups a day, take it in ½ cup amounts. For a chronic condition, you can take 1 cup at a time.

Dosages for children are much smaller. The following guidelines are based on an adult dose of 1 cup and the average weight for children's age groups. You will need to adjust accordingly. The smaller amounts are for the youngest in each age group. For example, in the dosage of 1 to 3 teaspoons, give a two-year-old 1 teaspoon and a four-year-old up to 3.

- Ages two to four—1 to 3 teaspoons a day
- Ages five to seven—1 to 3 tablespoons a day
- Ages eight to twelve—5 to 8 tablespoons a day

Use only the mildest herbs such as chamomile, lemon balm, and spearmint for small children. For the elderly, follow the adult dosage with adjustments for weight unless the person is frail or weak, in which case you may want to use the dosage for a seven-year-old. Regardless of age, if a person is on any type of medication, check with their physician before administering an herbal remedy.

Keep in mind that these are basic guidelines and the doses given throughout this book are suggestions. If an herb is not working for you, try a different one. Keep detailed notes when making and using remedies so you can adjust your recipes and dosages. Most of all, have fun and enjoy your work with herbs.

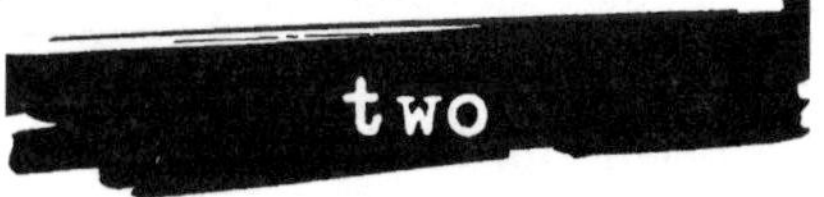

Basic Remedy Recipes and Applications

The amounts of herbs used in the recipes throughout this book are standard and regarded as a safe starting place for most people. As mentioned, when using an herb for the first time you may want to start with less. Because we are all unique, we may find that different amounts work better. As you prepare remedies, take notes to provide a marker for determining any adjustments that may be needed when making them again.

The recipes in this chapter and the next include amounts for both dried and fresh herbs to make it easy for you to use whichever you prefer. As you will notice, a smaller amount of dried herb is called for. This is because without its water content, an herb's flavor and potency are more concentrated.

When using seeds, lightly toast them first to enhance the flavor of your remedies. Place the seeds in a dry frying pan over low heat. Warm them just long enough to bring out their aroma. Crushing the seeds releases their oils. The easiest way to crush seeds is with a mortar and pestle. Use a circular motion as you press on the seeds. In a pinch, use the bottom edge of a small, heavy-duty pot or bowl. Place the seeds on a cutting board and press the pot or bowl back and forth over them.

A number of plants have multiple parts that can be used for remedies. When a specific part is required, the distinction will be made in the ingredients of a recipe. For example, "dandelion root" or "dandelion leaves" will be listed. In the case where either part can be used, the ingredient will be listed simply as "dandelion."

Tea/Tisane

Technically, "tea" is made only from the tea plant, *Camellia sinensis*, and marketed as black or green tea. An herbal tea is a mild infusion called a *tisane* (pronounced *tee-zahn*). The word *tisane* is from the thirteenth-century French *tisaine*, which was derived from the Latin *ptisana*.[4] Ptisana was a thin barley soup usually administered during illness because it was nourishing and easy to digest. However, because so many of us are used to calling a tisane *tea*, I have kept this convention throughout the book.

Tea can be made from various parts of plants: leaves, flowers, fruits, and seeds. As mentioned, seeds first need to be crushed. The difference between a tea and an infusion is that tea is made by the cup and consumed immediately, whereas infusions are made in larger amounts with some kept for later use. Also, an infusion is stronger because it is steeped longer.

4. Saberi, *Tea*, 26.

❁ Basic Tea Recipe

1–2 teaspoons dried herb, crumbled
or 3–4 teaspoons fresh herb, chopped
or 1 teaspoon tincture
1 cup water, boiled

Warm a cup or mug with hot tap water, empty it, and dry it. Add the herbs, and then carefully pour in the boiled water. When using fresh or dried herbs, cover and steep for 10 to 20 minutes before straining. When using a tincture, wait until the tea reaches a comfortable temperature before drinking.

Warming the cup before making tea keeps it from breaking and from drawing off some of the heat. Covering the cup helps keep tea warm, but it is more important for retaining the volatile oil in the herbs. The medicinal value comes from a plant's volatile or essential oil. These oils can be lost if the liquid is not covered while steeping. Special cups and mugs with fitted lids are available; however, placing a saucer over the top works just as well.

While tea is most often consumed warm or hot, depending on the situation and the herb, it can also be served at room temperature or chilled. The general course of treatment for many ailments is to drink 2 to 4 cups a day. When used as a sleep aid, drink tea at least thirty minutes before going to bed. When coping with a headache, drink tea several times throughout the day between meals.

Infusion

An infusion is usually made with the aerial parts of a plant: the leaves and flowers. Seeds are often used, too, and, as mentioned, they need to be crushed first. When making an infusion that will be ingested, toast the seeds to enhance their flavor. As with tea, an infusion should be covered while the herbs steep to retain the plant's volatile oils. A large jar, teapot, or French press can be used to steep an infusion. When using a teapot or French press, cover it with a dish towel to block the release of steam through the spout. This also helps keep the infusion warm. After straining out the herbs, an infusion can be stored in the refrigerator for a day or two and warmed as needed.

❁ Basic Infusion Recipe

4–6 tablespoons dried herb, crumbled
or 6–8 tablespoons fresh herb, chopped
1 quart water, boiled

Warm a large glass jar with hot tap water, empty it, and dry it. Add the herbs, and then carefully pour in the boiled water. Cover and steep for 30 to 45 minutes. Strain out the herbs before using or storing in the refrigerator.

When made for topical use, infusions can be stronger than those taken internally. Double the plant material or allow it to soak for several hours. Herbal infusions can be used in the bath for a therapeutic soak in the tub or to make other types of remedies such as an ointment and salve. They can also be used for other applications such as a compress and foot soak.

Cold Infusion

Also called a *maceration*, a cold infusion is made with cold water instead of hot. It uses the same amount of water and plant material as noted above. Cover and steep for twelve to twenty-four hours in a cool place. Strain out the herbs and use as you would an infusion made with hot water. While the decoction method is usually used for roots, a maceration works best for valerian root.

Decoction

Generally stronger than an infusion, a decoction is made with the tougher, more fibrous parts of plants: roots, bark, twigs, nuts, dried berries, and seeds. Leaves and flowers can also be used in a decoction; however, these should be added later in the preparation process as too much or prolonged heat can destroy their medicinal properties.

Like an infusion, a decoction can be prepared with fresh or dried herbs. Either way, the plant material must be chopped or broken into small pieces. Berries, seeds, and nuts should be crushed. Toasting seeds and nuts in a dry frying pan before crushing them enhances the flavor of remedies. A decoction should be stored in the refrigerator where it will keep for two or three days. As with an infusion, more plant material can be used when making a remedy for topical applications. A decoction can be administered hot or cold.

❁ Basic Decoction Recipe

4–6 tablespoons dried herb, crumbled or crushed
or 6–8 tablespoons fresh herb, chopped or crushed
1 quart water

Place the herbs and water in a saucepan and bring to a boil. Stir, cover, and reduce the heat to as low as possible. Simmer for 20 to 30 minutes or until the liquid is reduced by about half. Let the mixture cool to room temperature before straining into a glass jar with a tight-fitting lid. Store in the refrigerator.

Compress

A compress is one way that an infusion or decoction can be used topically. A compress can be applied warm or cool. A warm compress relaxes muscles and soothes aches and pains. It also relieves tension and increases blood circulation. A cool compress is used to treat bruises, strains, and sprains by reducing swelling and inflammation. It also reduces fevers and eases headaches.

After making an infusion or decoction, soak a washcloth in it, wring out the excess moisture, and then place it over the area that needs treatment. Freshen the cloth by dipping it in the infusion or decoction every five minutes or so.

Fomentation

Alternating the application of warm and cool compresses is a remedy called *fomentation*. It is used to manipulate the flow of blood in an area of the body. Start with a warm compress for about five to ten minutes to relax muscles and open capillaries. Follow immediately with a cool compress, which causes the muscles and capillaries to constrict and push blood out of the area. Leave the cool compress on for two to four minutes. Replace it with a fresh warm compress, which will open the capillaries again, bringing fresh blood into the affected area. Continue alternating the compresses for twenty to twenty-five minutes. This is especially helpful for treating low back pain, muscle strains, and kidney stones.

Infused Oil

As the name of this remedy implies, herbs are steeped in oil instead of water. While infused oils are commonly used for cooking, medicinal oils are usually made with more plant material to make them more potent. Infused oils are used for massage and bath oils and for making bath salts, salves, and ointments. While oils are used for their emollient qualities, many also have healing properties that can enhance remedies and boost the effectiveness of herbs.

Like an infusion made with water, an infused oil can be made by cold or hot methods. While cold infused oil is easier to make, the process takes longer. Hot infused oil is quicker to prepare and can be stored longer—sometimes up to a year. Olive oil is often a good choice as it rarely goes rancid. The hot method works best with the tougher parts of a plant: roots, fruit, nuts, and seeds.

Cold Infused Oil

As with many preparations, an infused oil can be made with fresh or dried herbs. When using fresh herbs, allow them to sit at room temperature for several hours until they wilt, which will reduce the water content. Reducing the moisture in fresh herbs helps avoid potential bacteria or mold growth.

❁ Basic Cold Infused Oil Recipe

¼ cup dried herb, crumbled or crushed
or ¾ cup fresh herb, chopped or crushed
2 cups oil

Place the herbs and oil in a glass jar with a tight-fitting lid. Gently poke around with a butter knife to release any air pockets. Leave the jar open for several hours to allow additional air to escape. After putting on the lid, gently swirl the contents of the jar. Place it out of direct light where it will stay at room temperature for 4 to 6 weeks. Strain the oil into a dark glass bottle or jar to store.

Hot Infused Oil

For this preparation, use a double boiler to keep the oil from overheating, which has a negative effect on the quality of the herbs. Check the bottom pot from time to time to make sure all the water has not boiled off. As mentioned in Chapter 1, if you don't have a double boiler, a large stainless-steel mixing bowl can be placed over a saucepan of water. You will need a lid to cover the mixing bowl and oven mitts to lift the bowl from the saucepan.

❁ Basic Hot Infused Oil Recipe

¼ cup dried herb, crumbled or crushed
or ¾ cup fresh herb, chopped or crushed
2 cups oil

Place the herbs and oil in a double boiler and cover. With the heat as low as possible, warm the oil for 30 to 60 minutes. Remove the pot from the heat and allow the oil to cool completely. Place a stainless-steel strainer lined with a piece of muslin cloth over a bowl to strain the oil. When it stops dripping, fold the cloth over the plant material and press to squeeze as much oil as possible from the herbs. Store the oil in a dark glass bottle or jar.

To make the straining process easier, place the herbs in a muslin bag before adding them to the double boiler. When the oil is completely cool, squeeze the bag to get as much oil as possible from the herbs.

Ointment, Salve, and Balm

These preparations are basically the same but differ in the amount of solidifier used to thicken them. An ointment is the least firm and has the advantage of being the easiest to apply. A salve has a firmer consistency and a balm is very firm to hard. These preparations absorb slowly and form a protective layer on the skin. In the following recipes, beeswax and cocoa butter are used as solidifiers. Beeswax forms more of a protective layer than cocoa butter, but it is worth experimenting to determine which one works best for you according to the ailment you are treating.

Making an ointment, salve, or balm is the second step in a two-step process; the first is to make an infused oil. The following recipes assume that the first step is complete. Because the consistency of a preparation depends on the ingredients, it is helpful to have a little extra infused oil, beeswax, or cocoa butter on hand in case you need to adjust your preparation. It is important to experiment and take notes so you can repeat a recipe or adjust it accordingly when you prepare it again.

Small amounts are used in the following recipes in order to have fresh remedies on hand. Preparing small amounts also makes it easy to quickly whip up a batch when you need it. I find it especially convenient to use small jars with screw-on lids because I can store the remedy in the same jar that I use to prepare it.

Beeswax is sold in blocks, bars, and pellets. The pellets are also called *pastilles*, *pearls*, and *beads*. Blocks of wax can be grated like hard cheese, which makes it easier to measure and melt. Pellets are convenient and easy to use but can be pricey. I find it economical to buy beeswax in 1-ounce bars, which is equal to 2 tablespoons. To measure smaller amounts, cut the bar in half for ½ ounce or in half again. To make it easier to cut, place the beeswax bar in a plastic bag and set it in a bowl of hot tap water for about ten to fifteen minutes. When you are ready to make a remedy, chop the beeswax into smaller pieces so it will melt faster.

❁ Basic Ointment, Salve, and Balm Recipe with Beeswax

½ ounce beeswax, chopped
4–10 tablespoons infused oil

Place the beeswax and infused oil in a glass jar, and then set it in a saucepan of water. Warm over low heat, stirring until the beeswax melts. Remove from the heat and allow the mixture to cool slightly. To test the consistency, spoon a little onto a plate and put it in the refrigerator for a couple minutes. If you want your preparation firmer, add a little more beeswax. If it is too thick, add a bit more infused oil. When you are happy with the consistency, let it cool completely before using or storing.

When working with oil and beeswax, it may be helpful to think and measure in ratios. An oil-to-beeswax ratio of 9:1 to 10:1 works well for an ointment, 6:1 to 8:1 for a salve, and 4:1 to 5:1 for a balm. Keep in mind that the consistency of your mixture depends on the viscosity of the oil you use. Don't worry if it is not quite what you want after the mixture has cooled and set because you can warm the jar in a saucepan of water and add a little more beeswax or infused oil. If you do this, don't forget to update your notes.

While the nut butters we buy for our morning toast have a soft, creamy texture, cocoa is a hard butter, but it is not as hard as beeswax. Cocoa butter is sold in blocks and can be grated like cheese. I find that scraping it with a paring knife is an easy way to prepare amounts for measuring. Unlike beeswax, cocoa butter melts at a lower temperature, but it needs to be heated twice and then refrigerated to give it a smooth consistency.

❁ Basic Ointment, Salve, and Balm Recipe with Cocoa Butter

1–3 tablespoons cocoa butter, grated
1–2 tablespoons infused oil

Boil a little water in a saucepan and remove it from the heat. Place the cocoa butter and infused oil in a glass jar, and then set it in the water. Stir until the butter melts. Carefully remove the jar from the water and allow the mixture to cool to room temperature. You may notice that it precipitates; particles or little lumps seem to float throughout the oil.

Boil the water again, remove it from the heat, and then place the jar in the water. Stir the mixture until the particles disappear. Remove the jar from the water, let the mixture cool slightly, and then place it in the refrigerator for 5 to 6 hours. After removing it from the fridge, let the mixture come to room temperature before using or storing.

Again, it may be helpful to think in terms of ratios. An oil-to-cocoa butter ratio of 1½:1 to 2:1 works for an ointment, 1:1 to 1:1½ for a salve, and 1:2 or 1:3 for a balm. Although a balm usually needs to be scraped up with a fingernail, it begins to melt on contact with the skin.

As with beeswax, experiment to find a consistency you like using your favorite oils. Occasionally, a preparation made with cocoa butter may have a slightly mottled appearance. Nothing is wrong; this is the nature of hard butters. While little particles may appear again after removing the preparation from the refrigerator, these will melt on contact with the skin.

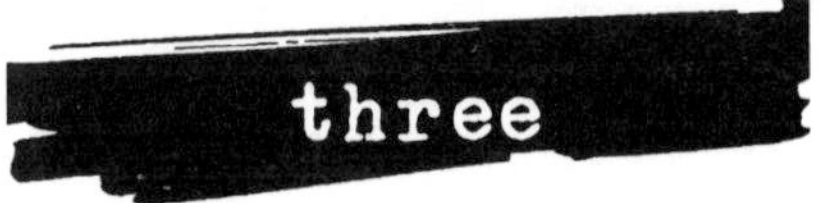

Additional Remedies and Applications

As in the previous chapter, these recipes include amounts for both dried and fresh herbs to help you use whichever you prefer. Some of the preparations covered in Chapter 2 serve as the base for several of the following remedies. Before storing, label your remedy with the date you prepared it, the herbs, and the other ingredients that you used to make it.

Gel

The base for a gel remedy comes from the aloe plant. Aloe vera is a familiar houseplant that is often kept in the kitchen for the first aid treatment of burns. Contained within the leaves, the gel is pale and translucent and has a slightly herby scent. Aloe vera boosts the power of herbs because it has antiseptic and antibacterial properties that work especially well for first-aid applications. It is also helpful for some other ailments.

While breaking off the tip of a leaf to treat a small burn is easy, you will need to cut up a large leaf to get enough gel to have an herbal remedy on hand. Having it ready-made is especially useful for taking along on day trips or summer vacation to treat sunburns, insect bites, and other minor mishaps.

An important thing to know about aloe leaves is that in addition to the translucent gel, a yellow juice called *bitter aloe* is exuded at the base of the leaves when they are cut. Bitter aloe is also found just under the skin of the leaves. Unlike the gel, it can be unpleasantly smelly and should not be used on the skin or ingested. Purchasing aloe gel is easier and more convenient. Refer to the aloe vera profile in Chapter 14 for details on what to look for when buying gel.

Like salves and ointments, preparing an aloe gel remedy is the second step in a two-step process. The first is to make an infusion, decoction, or infused oil. The following recipe assumes that the first step is complete.

❁ Basic Gel Recipe

3–4 tablespoons aloe vera gel

¼ cup infusion, decoction, or infused oil

Place the aloe gel in a bowl. With the infusion, decoction, or infused oil at room temperature, slowly combine with the gel until the mixture reaches a consistency you like. Gently stir until it is thoroughly mixed. Store in a glass jar with a tight-fitting lid.

Tincture

Stronger than an infusion or decoction, a tincture is made with alcohol instead of water or oil. Vodka, gin, brandy, and rum work well as a tincture base. Rum is particularly good to mask the taste of herbs, especially if they are a little bitter.

Methyl, isopropyl, and industrial alcohols should never be used to make a tincture.

Because a tincture is concentrated, it is administered in very small doses. It can be taken straight, or it can be used to make a medicinal syrup or tea. A tincture should not be used during pregnancy or by anyone with gastric inflammation.

❁ Basic Tincture Recipe

¾ cup dried herb, crumbled or crushed
or 1 ½ cups fresh herb, chopped or crushed
2 cups 80 to 100 proof alcohol

Place the herbs and alcohol in a glass jar with a tight-fitting lid. Close and shake for 1 to 2 minutes, and then set aside. Shake the jar every other day for 2 to 4 weeks before straining out the herbs. Store in a dark glass bottle away from sunlight.

A tincture will keep for up to two years. Another way to prepare it is to place enough dried herbs to fill ⅓ to ½ of a pint jar. When using fresh herbs, fill the jar to ¾ or slightly more. Pour in enough alcohol to cover the herbs and follow the directions as above.

A standard tincture dose is 1 teaspoon diluted in an ounce of water, tea, or fruit juice two or three times a day. If you don't like the alcohol, add 1 teaspoon of tincture to a cup of boiling water, and then wait about five minutes for the alcohol to evaporate. Tinctures can also be used straight by putting 10 to 15 drops under the tongue.

While it is not as potent, apple cider and apple cider vinegar can be substituted as a tincture base for anyone who prefers to avoid using alcohol. Cider or vinegar tinctures should steep for six weeks before straining out the herbs. A cider or vinegar tincture will keep for six to eight months. In addition to the standard methods of dosing, this type of tincture can be administered by sprinkling it on a salad.

Liniment

Like a tincture, a liniment is made with alcohol; however, it is for topical application only and should never be taken internally. A liniment is used to relieve the pain of stiff joints, sore muscles, strains, and sprains. It also aids in healing bruises and disinfecting wounds. A warming liniment can be made with cayenne to relieve pain and stiffness; a cooling liniment can be made with peppermint to reduce swelling and inflammation. To apply a liniment, rub it onto the affected area, or saturate a washcloth to use as a compress.

Isopropyl alcohol, also known as rubbing alcohol, is often recommended for a liniment base and is effective. However, alcohol can dry the skin, and for some people it can be a dermal irritant. Witch hazel serves as a good liniment base because it contains a low amount of alcohol—usually about 14 percent. Another alternative is to use witch hazel water and add a little isopropyl alcohol so you can control the amount of alcohol in the liniment. White vinegar can also be used as the base ingredient, although it is not as warming. When you label your liniment remedy, be sure to note that it is for external use only.

❁ Basic Liniment Recipe

4 tablespoons dried herb, crumbled or crushed
2 cups isopropyl alcohol, witch hazel, or white vinegar

Place the herbs and alcohol or other base ingredient in a glass jar with a tight-fitting lid. Close and shake for 1 or 2 minutes. Set aside for 4 to 6 weeks, giving the jar a good shake every day. Strain out the herbs, and then store in a dark glass bottle away from sunlight.

Poultice

A poultice is an herbal paste that is applied to an affected area. It can be used to ease muscle or nerve pain, insect bites, beestings, burns, and swollen glands. A poultice draws impurities out of infected wounds and boils. Like other remedies, it can be prepared with fresh or dried herbs. When treating a bruise, a poultice can be made with dried herbs and witch hazel instead of water.

❁ Basic Fresh Herb Poultice Recipe

½ cup fresh herb, chopped or crushed
1 cup water

Place the water in a saucepan. Mash the herbs as much as possible before adding them to the water. Stir and simmer on low heat for 1 to 3 minutes. Allow the mixture to cool to a comfortable temperature. Strain off the liquid.

❁ Basic Dried Herb Poultice Recipe

1–2 tablespoons dried herb, crumbled or crushed
water, enough to moisten

Boil a little water and add just enough to moisten the herbs and make a thick paste.

Whichever way you make it, when the poultice is cool enough to handle, cover the skin with gauze and spoon on a sufficient amount of herb paste to cover the affected area with a thick ¼- to ½-inch layer. Cover with another piece of gauze to keep the poultice in place. Cover the poultice with a towel to keep it warm for as long as possible. Remove it when it starts to cool. Apply a poultice one to three times a day, making a fresh one each time.

A poultice can be messy and depending on where you need to apply it, it can be a challenge. Following is an easier alternative using dried herbs to make and apply a poultice.

❁ Basic Easy Poultice Recipe

1–2 tablespoons dried herb, crumbled or crushed
2–3 cups water

Place the herbs in a muslin bag and set aside. Bring the water to a boil in a saucepan, and then remove it from the heat. Place the bag of herbs in the water for 1 to 3 minutes to moisten and warm the plant material. Remove from the water and press out excess moisture.

Check that the bag of herbs is not too hot, and then set it directly on the affected area. Cover the poultice with a towel to keep it warm for as long as possible, and then remove it when it starts to cool. As with the conventional method, apply a poultice one to three times a day, making a fresh one each time. If the area to treat is very small, use a tea filter bag to hold the herbs.

Powders and Capsules

Powdered herbs can be purchased, or you can make your own with dried herbs using a blender, food processor, or flour grinder. Store the powder in a glass jar with a tight-fitting lid away from sunlight.

Powders can be mixed into other preparations or taken in capsules, which is easier if you do not like the taste of a particular herb. Valerian is one such plant that many prefer to take in capsule form because of its taste and odor.

Gelatin and vegetarian-based capsule cases are available in many health food stores and online. The amount that each capsule can hold depends on the density of the powdered herb. Less of a coarsely ground powder will fit than one that is finely ground. Capsule size "1" holds between 300 and 600 milligrams, size "2" between 200 and 400 milligrams. It is important to begin with a minimal amount to determine what works best for you.

The most important thing to remember when filling capsules is that your hands must be completely dry, otherwise they will stick to your fingers. Capsules have two different halves: one is longer and slightly narrower (the bottom); the other is shorter and slightly wider (the cap), which fits over the bottom half. To fill, sprinkle a small mound of powdered herb on a saucer, and then scoop as much powder as you can into the bottom half of the capsule. Another way to fill them is to use a small piece of paper to make a tiny funnel so you can pour the powder into the bottom half. Either way, when you get as much as you can into the capsule, slide the halves together. Store capsules in a dark glass container with a tight-fitting lid in a cool, dry place.

Bath Salts

When used in the bath, herbs help relieve pain and stiffness. Salts contain minerals that aid in the release of toxins from the muscles and joints, which is beneficial when dealing with infectious illnesses, arthritis, and sore muscles. Bath salts also promote relaxation, which can ease stress and relieve nervous tension.

Commonly used as a base for bath salts, Epsom salt is healing in its own right. Named for the town in England where it was discovered, Epsom salt is a mineral compound that is helpful in relieving arthritis, bruises, inflammation, sore muscles, psoriasis, sprains, and strains. It can be purchased in grocery stores and pharmacies. Check that it is United States Pharmaceutical (USP) grade as this is high quality and suitable for personal care. Technical grade, also known as agricultural and industrial grade, is not for use in the home or on the body. Instead of Epsom salt for the base of this remedy, coarse sea salt can be used because it also contains healing minerals.

Preparing bath salts is the second step in a two-step process. The first is to make an infusion, decoction, or infused oil. The following recipe assumes that the first step is complete.

❁ Basic Bath Salts Recipe

2 cups Epsom or coarse sea salt
2 tablespoons baking soda (optional)
¾ cup infusion, decoction, or infused oil

Place the dry ingredients in a glass or porcelain bowl. Slowly add the infusion, decoction, or infused oil and stir until thoroughly mixed. Store in a glass jar with a tight-fitting lid.

The optional baking soda in the recipe helps soothe any inflammation and soften the skin. To use the salts, add a cup or two under the running tap to dissolve them.

Foot Soak

Infusions, decoctions, and bath salts can be used for a foot soak, which is also known as a footbath. Add a cup of bath salts or a quart of infusion or decoction to water in a basin. A warm or hot foot soak increases circulation, aids in healing a cold or flu, and helps deal with insomnia. Odd as it may seem, a foot soak can help relieve headaches, too, by drawing blood down to the feet and relieving pressure in the head. A cool footbath is a good perk-up on hot summer days when feet can be sweaty, swollen, and sore.

Medicinal Honey

As Mary Poppins told us, taking medicine is easier with a teaspoon of sugar, and honey is a good way to administer herbs, especially to children. Quite simply, it is an infusion made with honey instead of water or oil. There are two ways to make medicinal honey. The herbs can be crushed or chopped and put directly into the honey, or they can be placed in a small muslin bag for easy removal. Dry herbs placed directly into the honey can be strained out before storage or they can be left in. Fresh herbs should be removed before storage because of their water content, which can foster the growth of bacteria or mold.

❁ Basic Medicinal Honey Recipe

½ cup dried herb, crumbled or crushed
or ¾ cup fresh herb, chopped or crushed
1 cup honey

Pour the honey into a slightly larger jar, and then set it in a saucepan of water. Warm over low heat until the honey becomes less viscous. Add the herbs or place them in a muslin bag before adding to the honey. Use a butter knife to stir loose herbs throughout the honey or to push the bag of herbs down so it is completely covered. Continue warming for 15 to 20 minutes.

Remove from the heat and set aside until the honey is completely cool. Put the lid on the jar and store it out of direct light in a cupboard at room temperature for a week. To remove the herbs, heat the honey, and then strain it into another jar or remove the herb bag. Squeeze the herb bag to wring out as much honey as possible.

Medicinal honey can be stored in a cupboard for up to eighteen months. A spoonful of honey can be taken straight, or it can be used to sweeten tea.

Things to Know When Buying Honey

When purchasing honey, there are a number of things to keep in mind, especially for medicinal purposes. The words *pure* and *natural* on the label may sound good, but they are meaningless. Unlike the term *organic,* there is no government agency or other set of standards for these designations.

Honey can range from a very light golden color to dark mahogany. A good quality honey should be cloudy, not clear. This is due to the pollen content, which gives honey its valuable enzymes, vitamins, minerals, and antioxidants. The traditional filtering process catches wax, bee parts, and debris from the hive but leaves the pollen in the honey.

The best sources for good honey are local beekeepers or local farmers markets. If these are not available for you, try health food stores where you can often get locally sourced organic honey. You might also find it in a specialty section of a supermarket. As always, read labels carefully so you know exactly what you are getting.

Steam Inhalation

Along with steam, the antiseptic, antibacterial, and/or antiviral properties of some herbs help clear and soothe respiratory airways. Steam is a good way to treat congested sinuses, chest infections, colds, and the flu. In addition to relieving congestion, facial steams are good for the complexion because they deep clean the pores and add moisture to the skin.

❁ Basic Steam Inhalation Recipe

5–8 tablespoons dried herb, crumbled or crushed
or 6–10 tablespoons fresh herb, chopped or crushed
1 quart water

Place the water in a saucepan and bring to a boil. Add the herbs, cover, and simmer on low heat for 1 or 2 minutes. Remove the saucepan from the stove and place it on a table or countertop where you can easily access it.

Place a bath towel over your head to create a tent above the steaming water. Close your eyes and hold your face a comfortable distance from the water so the steam will not be too hot. Stay under the tent for three to five minutes or until the water is no longer steaming. If it feels too hot, lift the towel to allow cool air into the tent.

The combination of steam and herbs is also a good way to clean the air of a sickroom and to humidify or freshen a room in the winter. Place a steaming saucepan in the room where it is needed. When it cools, the mixture can be reheated to generate more steam.

Syrup

Syrup is a soothing treatment for sore throats and coughs. A dose is usually 1 teaspoon as needed. A syrup can be made with dried herbs or a tincture.

❁ Basic Syrup Recipe using Dried Herbs

8 tablespoons dried herbs, crumbled or crushed
1 quart water
1 cup honey

Combine the herbs and water in a saucepan, cover, and bring to a boil. Reduce the heat to as low as possible and simmer at least 30 minutes or until the volume is reduced by half. Strain out the herbs, return 2 cups of liquid to the saucepan, and add the honey. Warm on low heat, stirring until the mixture is smooth. Remove from the heat, allow the mixture to cool slightly, and then pour into a glass jar with a tight-fitting lid. Store in the refrigerator where it will keep for several weeks.

❁ Basic Syrup Recipe using a Tincture

2–4 tablespoons tincture
1 cup honey
½ cup water

Combine the honey and water in a saucepan. Warm over low heat, stirring until it has a smooth consistency. Add the tincture and mix thoroughly. Remove from the heat and pour into a glass jar with a tight-fitting lid. Allow the mixture to cool completely before putting the lid on. Store in the refrigerator where it will keep for up to 6 months.

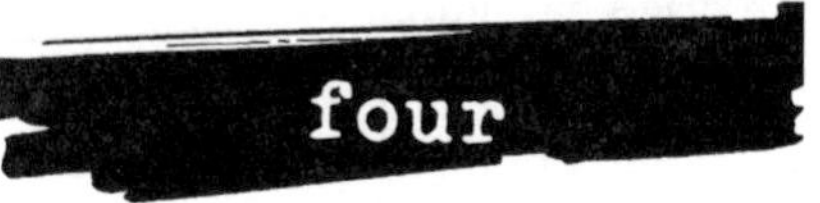

First Aid

This chapter covers ailments and injuries that require immediate attention or treatment that should not be delayed. Seek medical advice for any condition that worsens or becomes prolonged. The information presented here is not intended to take the place of a first aid course.

While some remedies need to be made fresh, others can be prepared ahead of time and stored. As you work with herbal remedies, you will be able to gauge how much to make and keep on hand to suit your needs.

Bruises

A bruise is an indication that there is bleeding underneath the skin. It is usually accompanied by swelling, tenderness, and discoloration that may change in color or intensity. Although a bruise goes away on its own, herbal remedies can be used to hasten the healing process while soothing minor pain. A large bruise that forms a lump is called a *hematoma*. Consult your doctor if bruising persists longer than five or six days or if it is accompanied by painful swelling.

❁ Bay, Parsley, and Witch Hazel Poultice

1 tablespoon dried bay laurel, crumbled
1 tablespoon dried parsley, crumbled
Witch hazel, enough to moisten

Combine the bay laurel and parsley in a small bowl. Add just enough witch hazel to moisten the herbs and make a thick paste.

To use: Cover the skin with gauze, and then spoon on enough of the poultice to cover the bruised area. Alternatively, place the poultice in a muslin bag and place it over the bruise. Use a piece of gauze to hold the poultice in place for about 10 minutes.

❁ Mullein and Yarrow Compress

5 tablespoons dried mullein, crumbled
5 tablespoons dried yarrow, crumbled
1 quart water, boiled

Pre-warm a large glass jar with hot tap water before adding the mullein, yarrow, and boiled water. Cover and steep for 40 to 45 minutes before straining.

To use: Soak and wring out a washcloth, and then place it over the bruise. Freshen the cloth by dipping it in the infusion every 5 minutes or so. Apply for about 20 minutes.

In a pinch, witch hazel can be used on its own and gently applied to the bruise with a cotton ball. Other herbs to use include burdock, caraway, fennel, hyssop, lavender, rosemary, St. John's wort, and thyme. Additional ingredients that help ease bruising are beeswax and olive oil.

Burns and Scalds

A burn is caused by dry heat, such as touching a hot stove. A scald is a burn caused by something wet, such as steam or hot water. Treatment for either type of burn is the same. There are three categories of burns. With a first-degree burn, the skin is red and unbroken. With a second-degree burn, the skin is red and blistered. A third-degree burn is more severe with the full depth of the skin involved and possibly charred. There is often little initial pain with a third-degree burn because the nerve endings have been damaged. Seek immediate professional medical attention for a third-degree burn. Also, go to the hospital immediately if you receive a chemical or electrical burn.

For a first- or second-degree burn or scald, begin treatment with cool or lukewarm water for about ten to fifteen minutes to bring down the temperature of the burn site. A wet compress can be used to cool the skin if clean running water is not available. Do not use ice or ice water as it can cause further damage to the skin and impede the healing process.

❁ Aloe and Mint Gel

For the infused oil:

3 teaspoons dried spearmint or peppermint, crumbled

¼ cup coconut oil

For the gel:
3–4 tablespoons aloe vera gel
¼ cup infused oil

Place the mint and coconut oil in a double boiler and cover. With the heat as low as possible, warm the oil for 45 minutes. Remove from the heat and allow the infused oil to cool completely before straining. Place the aloe vera in a bowl and slowly add the infused oil until the gel reaches a consistency you like. Gently stir until it is thoroughly mixed. Store in a glass jar with a tight-fitting lid.

To use: Apply a thin layer over the burn area several times a day.

❁ Lavender and St. John's Wort Ointment

For the infused oil:
1½ teaspoons dried lavender, crumbled
½ teaspoon dried St. John's wort, crumbled
¼ cup olive oil

For the ointment:
2 tablespoons cocoa butter, grated
¼ cup infused oil

Place the lavender, St. John's wort, and olive oil in a double boiler and cover. With the heat as low as possible, warm the oil for 30 to 40 minutes. Allow the infused oil to cool slightly before straining. Add the infused oil to a glass jar with the cocoa butter. Boil a little water in a saucepan and remove it from the heat. Place the jar in the water and stir until the cocoa butter melts. Remove the jar from the water and allow the mixture to cool to room temperature.

Small particles usually appear in the mixture as it cools. Boil the water again, place the jar in the water, and stir until the particles disappear. Remove the jar from the water, let the mixture cool slightly, and then place it in the refrigerator for 5 to 6 hours. Allow the ointment to come to room temperature before using or storing.

To use: Apply a thin layer to the burn area several times a day.

In addition to soothing pain, lavender and St. John's wort have antibacterial and antiseptic properties that can prevent infection. This ointment can be used for cuts, scratches, and abrasions, too. Both peppermint and spearmint are also antibacterial and help cool the skin. If you have an aloe vera plant, you can simply break a leaf open and apply some of the gel to a minor burn. Aloe will relieve pain and help prevent scarring. Other herbs and ingredients that can be used to treat a burn or scald include beeswax, chamomile, and hyssop.

Cuts and Abrasions

Caused by sharp objects or friction, minor cuts, scrapes, scratches, and abrasions can become infected if not promptly treated. After washing your hands, clean the area with warm water and gentle soap. For a cut or scratch that is bleeding, cover it with gauze and apply gentle pressure until it stops. Seek professional medical treatment for a wound that is bleeding profusely, involves an extensive area, or is caused by an animal.

❁ Yarrow and Mullein Wash

6 tablespoons dried yarrow, crumbled
5 tablespoons dried mullein, crumbled
1 quart water, boiled

Pre-warm a large glass jar with hot tap water, and then add the yarrow, mullein, and boiled water. Cover and steep for 30 to 35 minutes before straining.

To use: Place the infusion in a spray bottle to apply to the cut or abrasion or slowly pour it over the wound.

❁ Oregano and Nettle Salve

For the infused oil:
½ tablespoon dried oregano, crumbled
½ tablespoon dried nettle, crumbled
½ cup jojoba oil

For the salve:
½ ounce beeswax, chopped into small pieces
7–8 tablespoons infused oil

Place the oregano, nettle, and jojoba oil in a double boiler and cover. With the heat as low as possible, warm the oil for 40 to 45 minutes. Remove the infused oil from the heat and allow it to cool slightly before straining. Place the beeswax and infused oil in a glass jar in a saucepan of water. Warm over low heat, stirring until the beeswax melts. Remove from the heat and allow the mixture to cool completely before using or storing.

> ***To use:*** Apply to the affected area and cover with a bandage.

Yarrow is exceptional for stanching bleeding, numbing pain, and acting as an antiseptic. Nettle also has styptic properties to help stop bleeding. Mullein and oregano have antiseptic and antibacterial properties that fight infection.

Powdered cayenne can be used to stop bleeding and disinfect a cut or scratch. Just sprinkle a pinch of it over the wound. Yes, it will sting, but only for a moment, and it will stop the pain caused by the wound. The Lavender and St. John's Wort Ointment included under Burns and Scalds is also effective for cuts and abrasions. Additional herbs to use include angelica, chamomile, garlic, ginger, hyssop, rosemary, sage, thyme, and turmeric. Other ingredients that help clean and heal cuts and abrasions are aloe vera, olive oil, and witch hazel.

Fever

A fever is usually an indication that the body is fighting an infection. In addition to an elevated temperature, other symptoms can include sweating, chills, shivering, headache, weakness, and muscle aches. Call your doctor if an oral temperature reaches 103° F (39.4° C) for an adult and 100° F (37.8° C) for a child.

❁ Feverfew and Chamomile Compress

7 tablespoons dried feverfew, crumbled
5 tablespoons dried chamomile, crumbled
1 quart water, boiled

Pre-warm a large glass jar with hot tap water before adding the feverfew, chamomile, and boiled water. Cover and steep for 50 minutes before straining.

> ***To use:*** Soak and wring out a washcloth, and then lay it across the forehead. Applying the compress to the neck and armpits also helps. Freshen the cloth every 5 minutes or so. Apply for 20 minutes.

❁ Lemon Balm and Hyssop Infusion

4 tablespoons dried lemon balm, crumbled
2 tablespoons dried hyssop, crumbled
1 quart water, boiled

Pre-warm a large glass jar with hot tap water, and then add the lemon balm, hyssop, and boiled water. Cover and steep for 30 minutes before straining.

> ***To use:*** Drink ½ cup every 2 hours over a 6-hour period. Drink the infusion cool or at room temperature.

Lemon balm and hyssop encourage sweating, which helps break a fever. In addition to the above measures, be sure to keep hydrated. Other herbs that can be used to bring down a fever include angelica, anise, coriander, fennel, ginger, lemongrass, nettle, peppermint, sage, spearmint, and yarrow.

Hangover

A hangover involves a group of symptoms that can include headache, nausea, vomiting, muscle aches, fatigue, sensitivity to light and sound, and dizziness. While the passage of time is the only thing that cures a hangover, staying hydrated and sleeping help ease the symptoms.

❁ Dandelion Tea

1½ teaspoons dried dandelion leaves, crumbled
1 cup water, boiled

Pre-warm a cup or mug with hot tap water before adding the dandelion and boiled water. Cover and steep for 10 minutes, and then strain.

> ***To use:*** Drink several cups throughout the day. Honey can be added for taste.

❁ Cayenne and Tomato Juice

8 ounces tomato or V8 juice
1 pinch cayenne, powdered

Add the cayenne to the tomato or V8 juice, stir, and drink.

Known for clearing nasal congestion, cayenne also helps clear a hungover head. The classic hangover cure of tomato juice helps the body deal with alcohol and aids in hydration.

A strong tea made with thyme can also help. A cool compress over the eyes or forehead while resting is soothing, too.

Insect Bites and Beestings

Whether playing or working outdoors, encountering bees and insects is inevitable, and no matter how careful we may be, at some point we will get stung or bitten. Symptoms include redness, pain, itching, and swelling. Wash the bite or sting site with soap and water. When stung by a bee, try to pull out the stinger as soon as possible.

A severe allergic reaction called *anaphylaxis* is marked by trouble breathing. Other symptoms can include a feeling of tightness in the chest and/or throat and faintness. It can occur within minutes or an hour of being stung or bitten. Call 911 and use an EpiPen immediately, if one is available.

❁ Basil and Lemongrass Salve

For the infused oil:
½ tablespoon dried basil, crumbled
½ tablespoon dried lemongrass, crumbled
½ cup olive oil

For the salve:
½ ounce beeswax, chopped into small pieces
7–8 tablespoons infused oil

Place the basil, lemongrass, and olive oil in a double boiler and cover. With the heat as low as possible, warm the oil for 30 to 40 minutes. Remove from the heat, allow the infused oil to cool slightly, and then strain. Place the beeswax and infused oil in a glass jar in a saucepan of water. Warm over low heat, stirring until the beeswax melts. Remove from the heat and allow the mixture to cool completely before using or storing.

To use: Apply several times a day or as needed.

❁ Nettle, Peppermint, and Aloe Gel

For the infused oil:
2 teaspoons dried nettle leaves, crumbled
1 teaspoon dried peppermint, crumbled
¼ cup coconut oil

For the gel:
3–4 tablespoons aloe vera gel
¼ cup infused oil

Place the nettle, peppermint, and coconut oil in a double boiler and cover. With the heat as low as possible, warm for 35 to 40 minutes. Remove from the heat and allow the infused oil to cool completely before straining. Place the aloe in a bowl and slowly add the infused oil until the gel reaches a consistency you like. Gently stir until it is thoroughly mixed. Store in a glass jar with a tight-fitting lid.

To use: Apply several times a day or as needed.

The antihistamine properties of basil and nettle relieve the swelling and itching of stings and bites. In fact, if you have basil in your garden, you can start treating a bite or sting before going indoors by crushing and rubbing a leaf onto the affected area. Basil is especially effective for wasp stings and mosquito bites. The anti-inflammatory properties of beeswax, coconut oil, and olive oil make effective remedy bases.

A poultice using any of the herbs mentioned here also works well. In a pinch, plain witch hazel eases the itching and swelling, especially if it is cold. Keep a bottle of witch hazel in the fridge during the summer months for quick relief. Other herbs and ingredients to use for insect bites and beestings include bay laurel, black cohosh, chamomile, fennel, jojoba oil, lavender, lemon balm, mullein, parsley, sage, spearmint, and St. John's wort.

Poison Ivy, Poison Oak, and Poison Sumac

All three of these plants secrete an oil called *urushiol*, which can be found on their leaves, stems, and roots. Touching the plant with your hands increases the risk of spreading the oil to other parts of the body. It can also be transferred from clothing, pets, and anything that came into contact with the plant. The oil usually causes an allergic reaction in the form of a rash, which is not contagious. Symptoms include swelling, itching, redness, and blisters. They can appear within twelve hours or two days after contact with the oil. The first line of defense is to wash your hands and all exposed skin with lukewarm soapy water as soon as possible after contact.

See your doctor immediately or go to the hospital if you have inhaled the smoke from burning any of these plants because it can cause a severe allergic reaction that includes difficulty breathing. Also see your doctor if symptoms don't improve, if they worsen, or if you develop a fever of 100° F (37.8° C).

❁ Burdock Poultice

2 tablespoons dried burdock root, finely chopped
2–3 cups water

Place the burdock in a muslin bag and set aside. Bring the water to a boil in a saucepan, and then remove it from the heat. Place the bag of burdock in the water for 2 to 3 minutes to moisten and warm the plant material. Remove from the water and press out excess moisture.

> ***To use:*** First wash the affected area with soapy water and apply witch hazel. Check that the bag of herbs is not too hot, and then set it directly on the affected area. Cover it with a towel to keep the poultice warm for as long as possible. Remove when it starts to cool.

❁ Aloe and Burdock Gel

For the infused oil:
3 teaspoons dried burdock root, chopped
¼ cup coconut oil

For the gel:
4 tablespoons aloe vera gel
¼ cup infused oil

Place the burdock and coconut oil in a double boiler and cover. With the heat as low as possible, warm for 45 minutes. Remove from the heat and allow the infused oil to cool completely before straining. Place the aloe in a bowl and slowly add the infused oil until the gel reaches a consistency you like. Stir until it is thoroughly mixed. Store in a glass jar with a tight-fitting lid.

To use: After washing the affected area with soapy water and applying witch hazel, use a liberal amount of gel several times a day or as needed.

In a pinch, plain witch hazel or aloe vera gel soothes the itching as does a compress prepared with plain cool water. Be sure to wash the clothes and shoes you were wearing and any gear you were carrying when you came into contact with the poison ivy, poison oak, or poison sumac. While pets are protected by their fur, they should be bathed in warm water with a mild de-greasing soap such as Dawn dish soap to remove the oil.

Sprains and Strains

A sprain is the stretching or tearing of a ligament, which is the fibrous tissue that connects two bones. A strain is the stretching or tearing of a muscle. Sprains are accompanied by pain, swelling, bruising, and limited range of motion. They most commonly occur in the ankles and wrists. Strains are accompanied by pain, swelling, muscle spasms, and the limited ability to move. They most often occur in the lower back and the back of the thighs. The first course of action is to put ice on the site of the sprain or strain. If ice is not available, apply a cold compress.

❁ Rosemary and Chamomile Compress

6 tablespoons dried rosemary, crumbled
6 tablespoons dried chamomile, crumbled
1 quart water, boiled

After pre-warming a large glass jar with hot tap water, add the rosemary, chamomile, and boiled water. Cover and steep for 45 to 50 minutes before straining. Place in the refrigerator for a few minutes to chill.

> ***To use:*** Soak and wring out a washcloth, and then place it over the area that needs treatment. Apply for 20 to 30 minutes, freshening the compress every 5 minutes or so. Use a compress several times a day, especially the first day. After the swelling has gone down in 2 or 3 days, apply warm compresses.

❁ Oregano and Bay Liniment

1½ tablespoons dried oregano, crumbled
1 tablespoon dried bay laurel, crumbled
1 cup witch hazel

Combine the oregano, bay laurel, and witch hazel in a glass jar with a tight-fitting lid. Close and shake for 1 or 2 minutes. Set aside for 4 to 6 weeks, giving the jar a good shake every day. Strain into a dark glass bottle.

> ***To use:*** Gently massage the affected area until it feels warm.

If you don't have a liniment on hand, an herbal infusion with olive oil can be used to gently massage the area. Witch hazel on its own also helps reduce inflammation. For muscle strains, a fomentation helps. Other herbs that can be used to relieve a strain or sprain include lavender, lemongrass, nettle, peppermint, St. John's wort, thyme, valerian, and yarrow.

Sunburn

A few hours after exposure to the ultraviolet (UV) light in the sun's rays, a sunburn can develop. Symptoms include pain, redness, and the surface of the skin feeling hot to the touch. It doesn't take a bright, sunny day to get a sunburn—it can occur on overcast days and from sunlamps. The first step in treatment is to cool the skin. While a cool shower helps, an herbal spray can cool the skin and aid in healing any damage. In some cases, a spray works best as a treatment because sunburn can be too painful to touch with an ointment or salve.

❁ Spearmint and Lavender Spray

5 teaspoons dried spearmint, crumbled
3 teaspoons dried lavender, crumbled
2 cups water, boiled

Pre-warm a large glass jar with hot tap water, and then add the spearmint, lavender, and boiled water. Cover and steep for 30 to 40 minutes before straining. Allow the infusion to cool to room temperature.

To use: Pour into a spray bottle with a fine mist setting and spray onto affected areas. Repeat several times a day or as needed.

❁ Chamomile and St. John's Wort Ointment

For the infused oil:
2 teaspoons dried chamomile, crumbled
½ teaspoon dried St. John's wort, crumbled
¼ cup jojoba oil

For the ointment:
2 tablespoons cocoa butter, grated
¼ cup infused oil

Place the St. John's wort, chamomile, and jojoba oil in a double boiler and cover. With the heat as low as possible, warm for 1 hour. Remove the infused oil from the heat and cool slightly before straining. Combine the infused oil and cocoa butter in a glass jar. Boil a little water in a saucepan and remove it from the heat. Place the jar in the water and stir until the cocoa butter melts. Remove it from the water and allow the mixture to cool to room temperature. Small particles usually appear in the mixture as it cools. Boil the water again, place the jar in the water, and stir until the particles disappear. Remove the jar from the water, let the mixture cool slightly, and then place it in the refrigerator for 5 to 6 hours. Allow the ointment to come to room temperature before using or storing.

To use: Gently apply several times a day.

The anti-inflammatory properties of the ingredients in the spray and ointment soothe and heal sun-damaged skin. Cocoa butter and jojoba oil also moisturize the skin. Aloe vera gel or a compress made with plain cool water can be used to relieve pain and discomfort. Other herbs and ingredients that help heal sunburned skin include beeswax, coconut oil, olive oil, peppermint, rosemary, and witch hazel.

Toothache

A toothache can result from a variety of reasons including a cavity, lost filling, broken tooth, and gum infection. Because a toothache seems to always occur at night or over the weekend when our dentists are not available, it is helpful to have something in the kitchen to use for relief until you can get an appointment. The first step for dealing with a toothache is to rinse the affected area with warm saltwater made with ½ teaspoon of salt in a cup of water.

❁ Ginger Mouthwash

¼ cup fresh ginger, chopped
2 cups water

Place the ginger and water in a saucepan and bring to a boil. Reduce the heat, cover, and simmer for 20 minutes. Let it cool to a comfortable temperature, and then strain.

To use: Take a little of the liquid in your mouth and tilt your head to hold it in the area of the aching tooth. Spit out and repeat until the mouthwash is gone.

❁ Thyme Compress

6 tablespoons dried thyme, crumbled
2 cups water, boiled

After pre-warming a glass jar with hot tap water, add the thyme and boiled water. Cover and steep for 1 hour before straining.

To use: Warm the mixture slightly, soak a gauze pad in the infusion, and then place it over the tooth. Freshen the pad by dipping it in the infusion every 5 minutes or so. Apply for about 20 minutes.

In a pinch, a tea bag can be used as a poultice to put herbs where you need them. Warm a chamomile, spearmint, or peppermint tea bag in hot water for two to three minutes. Make sure it is not too hot before gently placing it in your mouth over the tooth.

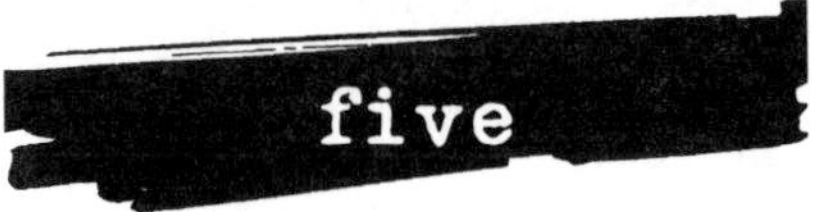

The Head, Ears, Eyes, Mouth, and Throat

Unlike the following chapters that focus on specific systems of the body, this one deals with ailments by their location. The head is a unique part of the body because it houses an array of sensory organs as well as the command center, the brain. It also contains a few parts of other systems, such as the mouth and nose.

Earache

While it often starts with an infection, an earache can have other causes such as a buildup of wax or water inside the ear. Wind, the common cold, allergies, and clenching or grinding the teeth can also cause ear pain. The pain can be sharp or dull, constant or fluctuating. Although earaches are more common in children, adults can get them, too.

❁ **Chamomile and Thyme Poultice**

6 tablespoons dried chamomile, crumbled
4 tablespoons dried thyme, crumbled
2–3 cups water

Place the chamomile and thyme in a muslin bag and set aside. Bring the water to a boil in a saucepan, and then remove it from the heat. Place the bag of herbs in the water for 2 to 3 minutes to moisten and warm the plant material. Remove from the water and press out excess moisture.

> ***To use:*** Check that the bag of herbs is not too hot, and then place it over the ear and surrounding area. Cover it with a towel to keep the poultice warm for as long as possible. Remove when it starts to cool.

❁ Feverfew Compress

¾ cup dried feverfew, crumbled
1 quart water, boiled

Pre-warm a large glass jar with hot tap water, and then add the feverfew and boiled water. Cover and steep for 1 hour before straining.

> ***To use:*** Warm the infusion to a comfortable temperature, soak and wring out a washcloth, and then place it over the ear and surrounding area. Freshen the cloth by dipping it in the infusion every 5 minutes or so. Apply for about 20 minutes.

The moist heat and anti-inflammatory properties of the herbs relieve discomfort and can help you cope with more severe pain until you can get to your doctor to treat the underlying cause. The compress also helps keep the head, ears, and neck warm. When caused by infection, adding garlic to the diet aids healing. Lavender and mullein can also be used to make a poultice or compress.

Eyes

Nowadays we spend so much time staring at computers, smartphones, and a wide range of electronic screens that it is no wonder our eyes get tired and irritated. Allergies, hay fever, colds, and the flu can also cause discomfort.

Puffy Eyes

Puffiness is the result of excessive fluid in the tissue around the eyes. It can be caused by allergies, sinus problems, fatigue, lack of sleep, hangover, stress, and dehydration.

❁ Fennel Compress

1 cup fresh fennel leaves, chopped
1 quart water

Place the fennel and water in a saucepan, cover, and simmer for 15 minutes. Let the mixture steep for 1 hour before straining. Place in the refrigerator for a few minutes to chill.

> ***To use:*** When the infusion is comfortably chilled, soak and wring out a washcloth, and then place it over the eyes as you rest for at least 10 minutes.

In a pinch, soak a couple chamomile tea bags in water, chill in the refrigerator for a few minutes, and then place them over the eyes as you rest. Parsley and rosemary can also be used to soothe puffy, irritated eyes. More than a quintessential beauty magazine tip, cucumber slices also work.

Sties and Chalazia

A bump at the edge of the eyelid or the base of an eyelash could be a stye or a chalazion. Known medically as a hordeolum, a stye is caused by a localized infection and is usually painful. A chalazion is a clogged oil gland that does not cause pain. While most sties and chalazia go away on their own within a couple days, herbs can speed them along and relieve discomfort.

❁ Thyme Tea

4 teaspoons dried thyme, crumbled
1 cup water, boiled

Pre-warm a cup or mug with hot tap water, and then add the thyme and boiled water. Cover and steep for 20 to 25 minutes before straining.

> ***To use:*** Warm the tea slightly, but make sure it is not too hot. Dip a cotton swab in the tea and carefully apply it to the stye or chalazion. Apply 2 or 3 times a day.

❁ Coriander Compress

5 tablespoons coriander seeds, crushed
2 cups water, boiled

Pre-warm a glass jar with hot tap water. Crush the coriander seeds, and then add them to the jar with the boiled water. Cover and steep for 1 hour, and then strain.

To use: Warm the mixture slightly, soak a gauze pad in the infusion, and then place it over the stye or chalazion. Freshen the pad by dipping it in the infusion every 5 minutes or so. Apply for about 15 minutes, 2 or 3 times a day.

Other herbs that can be used to treat sties and chalazia include burdock, chamomile, and turmeric. Keep in mind that turmeric will temporarily stain the skin when used topically.

Head Lice

As their name implies, *Pediculus capitis* live on the head. Spread by person-to-person contact, adult lice make their home on the scalp and feed on blood. While they do not carry infectious diseases, it is important to get rid of the lice and their eggs, which they attach to the hair shafts. The eggs are called *nits*. Over time, lice multiply exponentially. If left untreated, the inevitable scratching in response to the itching they cause can break the skin and lead to infection and other complications.

❁ Anise and Lemongrass Infusion

2 tablespoons aniseeds, crushed
1 tablespoon dried lemongrass, crumbled
1 cup coconut oil

Crush the aniseeds. Place them with the lemongrass and coconut oil in a double boiler and cover. With the heat as low as possible, warm for 1 hour. Allow the mixture to cool completely before straining.

> ***To use:*** You will need a shower cap and nit comb. A nit comb is a very fine-toothed comb available at pharmacies. Massage the infusion into the scalp and work it through the hair. Cover with the shower cap and leave on for the better part of a day or overnight. After removing the shower cap, carefully comb through the hair to remove the nits. Shampoo thoroughly. Repeat the treatment in a day or two. Use the nit comb on wet hair every 2 or 3 days for up to 2 weeks until you no longer find nits.

It is important to wash and carefully check combs, brushes, hair accessories, hats, scarves, clothes, and bed pillows for lice and their eggs. Other herbs that can be used to treat a head lice infestation are lavender, parsley, and thyme.

Headache

Headaches are one of the most common medical complaints. They are classified into two categories: primary and secondary. Primary headaches are not caused by other conditions; secondary headaches have an underlying cause. Common types of primary headaches include migraines, tension headaches, and cluster headaches. Cluster headaches occur for short periods several times throughout the day. Secondary headaches have a wide range of causes including concussion, dehydration, the common cold, the flu, hangover, panic attack, and sometimes serious conditions.

❁ Lavender and Chamomile Compress

6 tablespoons dried lavender, crumbled
6 tablespoons dried chamomile, crumbled
1 quart water, boiled

Pre-warm a large glass jar with hot tap water, and then add the lavender, chamomile, and boiled water. Cover and steep for 1 hour before straining.

> ***To use:*** Have the infusion at room temperature or place it in the refrigerator for a few minutes to slightly chill. Soak and wring out a washcloth, and then place it across the forehead while you rest. Freshen the cloth every 5 minutes or so.

❁ Ginger and Peppermint Massage Oil

3 tablespoons fresh ginger, coarsely grated
2 tablespoons dried peppermint, crumbled
2 cups jojoba oil

Place the ginger and jojoba oil in a double boiler and cover. With the heat as low as possible, warm the oil for 40 minutes. Remove from the heat, stir in the peppermint, and cover. Steep for 15 minutes before straining. Allow the oil to cool completely before using or storing.

> ***To use:*** Place a little oil on your fingertips and gently massage your temples and neck. Also try the pressure point used in traditional Chinese medicine: With your thumb on the palm side and index finger on the top side of the opposite hand, find the space at the base of the webbing between the thumb and index

finger. Press and hold for several minutes, and then firmly massage in a circular motion. Repeat on the other hand.

Lemon balm tea can also bring relief. Let it steep until cool, and then drink a cup at a time three times throughout the day. Black cohosh is effective for hormone-related headaches and St. John's wort for tension headaches. A foot soak with warm water or a warm infusion also helps by drawing blood down to the feet and relieving pressure in the head. Other herbs to use for a headache include angelica, basil, cayenne, coriander, dill, feverfew, lemongrass, oregano, parsley, rosemary, sage, thyme, turmeric, and valerian.

Migraine

There are headaches and then there are migraines. Excruciatingly painful, a migraine may be accompanied by symptoms such as throbbing pain, nausea, blurred vision, and visual disturbances called *auras*, which are often kaleidoscopic color patterns. Noise, light, and strong odors can aggravate a migraine. An ocular or aura migraine, which is also known as a silent migraine, is mainly characterized by visual disturbances with minor pain. The visual effects tend to last about twenty minutes.

❁ Feverfew Tea

4 teaspoons dried feverfew, crumbled
2 cups water, boiled

Pre-warm a large mug or glass jar with hot tap water, and then add the feverfew and boiled water. Cover and steep for 15 minutes before straining.

> ***To use:*** Drink a cup, and then take 2 to 3 tablespoons every 3 hours.

❁ Lemon Balm and Rosemary Infusion

- 4 tablespoons dried lemon balm, crumbled
- 2 tablespoons dried rosemary, crumbled
- 1 quart water, boiled

Pre-warm a large glass jar with hot tap water, and then add the lemon balm, rosemary, and boiled water. Cover and steep for 30 to 35 minutes before straining. Store in the refrigerator.

> ***To use:*** Warm and drink a cup at a time. Drink several times a day between meals.

Feverfew is especially helpful when consumed at the first sign of a migraine. A pinch of powdered cayenne dissolved in hot water taken at the onset may not completely eliminate a migraine, but it may bring some relief. After taking this remedy, follow it with a little milk to cool the mouth. Black cohosh is effective for hormone-related migraines. Try an herbal compress on the forehead, temples, or back of the neck. A cool compress for the eyes or just resting the eyes can ease a silent migraine. Other herbs to use for migraines include lavender, oregano, peppermint, thyme, and valerian.

The Mouth

Although the mouth is part of the gastrointestinal tract, its ailments are unique from the rest of the digestive system. It is also an integral part of the respiratory system.

Canker Sores

Also known as an aphthous ulcer and mouth ulcer, a canker sore is a small lesion in the mouth that is usually caused by friction or other irritation. The sore is white in the center and red around the edges. Canker sores sometimes occur in clusters of two or three. Although they usually clear up in a week or two on their own, canker sores can be annoying and are often painful.

❁ Rosemary Mouthwash

1½ teaspoons dried rosemary, crumbled
1 cup water, boiled

Pre-warm a cup or mug with hot tap water before adding the rosemary and boiled water. Cover and steep for 20 to 25 minutes, and then strain.

To use: Take half a mouthful, swish it around, and then hold it over the problem area. Spit out and repeat until the mouthwash is gone. Use several times a day.

❁ Sage and Thyme Poultice

¼ teaspoon dried sage, crumbled
¼ teaspoon dried thyme, crumbled
1 cup water, boiled

Place the sage and thyme in a tea filter bag. You may want to adjust the amount of herbs so that the tea bag will not be uncomfortably large to place in your mouth. Securely tie the tea bag shut, and then place it in a pre-warmed mug. Add the boiled water and allow the tea bag to warm for a couple minutes. Press out excess water.

To use: Make sure the tea bag is not too hot before placing it in your mouth over the canker sore. Leave it in place until it begins to cool. Repeat a couple times a day, making a fresh poultice each time.

The antiseptic and anti-inflammatory properties of rosemary, sage, and thyme help soothe and heal canker sores. In a pinch, if you have a box of chamomile tea bags, use one as a poultice. Warm it in a mug of boiled water for a few minutes and make sure it is not too hot before placing on the canker sore. Other herbs that can be used include basil, coriander, and mullein.

Cold Sores

Also known as a fever blister, a cold sore can occur almost anywhere on the body but most often appears just outside the mouth or on the lips. These blistering sores are caused by the herpes simplex virus (HSV-1), which is different from the genital herpes virus (HSV-2).

Other cold sore symptoms include tingling and itching. Often occurring in clusters, the blisters may ooze fluid and crust over. An outbreak can be triggered by a cold, the flu, stress, and fatigue. Cold sores can be spread by person-to-person contact.

❁ St. John's Wort Tincture

¾ cup dried St. John's wort leaves, crumbled
2 cups 80 to 100 proof alcohol (vodka, gin, brandy, or rum)

Place the St. John's wort and alcohol in a glass jar with a tight-fitting lid. Close and shake for 1 to 2 minutes. Set aside for 2 to 3 weeks, shaking the jar every other day. Strain and store in a dark glass bottle.

To use: Place a few drops on a cotton swab, and then dab it on the cold sore. Apply up to 3 times a day.

❁ Ginger and Lavender Salve

For the infused oil:
3 teaspoons fresh ginger, coarsely grated
2 teaspoons dried lavender, crumbled
½ cup jojoba oil

For the salve:
½ ounce beeswax, chopped into small pieces
7–8 tablespoons infused oil

Place the ginger and jojoba oil in a double boiler and cover. With the heat as low as possible, warm for 30 minutes. Remove from the heat and stir in the lavender. Cover and steep for 20 minutes before straining. Place the beeswax and infused oil in a glass jar in a saucepan of water. Warm over low heat, stirring until the beeswax melts. Remove from the heat and allow the mixture to cool completely before using or storing.

To use: Apply to the affected area several times a day.

If you don't have a tincture or salve on hand when an outbreak occurs, make a strong tea with any of the herbs mentioned here and use a cotton swab to dab it on the cold sore. Drinking 3 to 4 cups of lemon balm tea a day at the first indication of a cold sore helps prevent or reduce its severity. Coconut oil also helps soothe and heal a cold sore.

Gingivitis

Gingivitis is the inflammation, irritation, and redness of the gums around the base of the teeth. Other symptoms can include gum tenderness, bad breath, and bleeding. Usually caused by the lack of good oral care, gingivitis can lead to more serious gum disease and tooth loss.

❁ Basil and Spearmint Mouthwash

1 teaspoon dried basil, crumbled
1 teaspoon dried spearmint, crumbled
¾ teaspoon table salt
1 cup water, boiled

Pre-warm a cup or mug with hot tap water before adding the basil, spearmint, salt, and boiled water. Cover and steep for 20 minutes, and then strain.

To use: Take half a mouthful, swish it around, and then hold it over the problem area. Spit out and repeat until the mouthwash is gone. Use several times a day.

❁ Sage Tooth Powder

2 tablespoons dried sage, powdered
2 tablespoons baking soda

Combine the sage and baking soda in a small bowl and mix well. Store in a glass jar with a tight-fitting lid.

To use: Place a little of the mixture in the palm of your hand, wet your toothbrush, and dip it in the powder. Brush gently, especially around the gumline.

The astringent and anti-inflammatory properties of the herbs in these recipes help soothe any discomfort and reduce swelling. Baking soda neutralizes acids that contribute to gum disease. Along with sage, it also whitens teeth. Other herbs that can be used for gingivitis include lemongrass, mullein, peppermint, thyme, and turmeric. In addition to improving oral care and using herbal remedies, it is important to visit your dentist regularly.

Halitosis

Halitosis, or bad breath, happens to everyone at some point. Eating certain foods such as garlic, onions, and cabbage can cause bad breath. Tobacco and alcohol are also culprits. Other causes include the buildup of bacteria due to poor dental hygiene, a cavity, gum disease, and throat or sinus infection.

❁ Cilantro Tea

2–3 tablespoons fresh cilantro (coriander) leaves, chopped
1 cup water

Place the cilantro and water in a saucepan, cover, and bring to a boil. Reduce the heat and simmer for 2 to 3 minutes. Remove from the heat and steep for 10 minutes before straining.

To use: Drink or use as a mouthwash.

❁ Anise and Peppermint Mouthwash

3 tablespoons aniseeds, crushed
2 tablespoons dried peppermint, crumbled
1 quart water, boiled

Lightly toast the aniseeds in a dry frying pan over low heat before crushing. Pre-warm a glass jar with hot tap water, and then add the aniseeds, peppermint, and boiled water. Cover and steep for 40 minutes before straining.

To use: After brushing your teeth, take half a cup of the mouthwash and swish it around in your mouth before spitting out. Store the remaining infusion in the refrigerator.

Chewing a few aniseeds will also freshen the breath, especially after eating garlic. More than a simple dinner plate garnish, a little fresh parsley after a meal sweetens and clears the breath, too. Other herbs to use for halitosis include basil, caraway, dill, rosemary, sage, spearmint, thyme, and turmeric.

Temporomandibular Joint (TMJ) Pain

Acting like a sliding hinge, the temporomandibular joints (TMJ) connect the jawbone to the skull. Pain that occurs in either or both joints can be caused by clenching or grinding the teeth, arthritis, injury, genetics, stress, or a combination of factors. Referred pain can occur in the face, ears, and neck. TMJ issues can also cause headaches.

❁ Lavender and St. John's Wort Massage Oil

3 tablespoons dried lavender, crumbled
2 tablespoons dried St. John's wort, crumbled
2 cups coconut oil

Place the lavender, St. John's wort, and coconut oil in a double boiler and cover. With the heat as low as possible, warm the oil for 35 to 45 minutes. Remove from the heat and allow it to cool completely before straining.

> ***To use:*** Place a little oil on your fingertips and gently massage the temporomandibular joints and any area of referred pain.

❁ Coriander and Rosemary Compress

⅓ cup coriander seeds, crushed
⅓ cup dried rosemary, crumbled
1 quart water, boiled

Pre-warm a glass jar with hot tap water. Crush the coriander seeds, and then add them to the jar with the rosemary and boiled water. Cover and steep for 1 hour before straining.

To use: Warm to a comfortable temperature, soak and wring out a washcloth, and then place it over the painful area. Freshen the cloth every 5 minutes or so. Apply for 20 minutes.

Oregano can also be used for a warm compress or massage oil. A cup of valerian tea before bed helps relax muscles and ease TMJ pain.

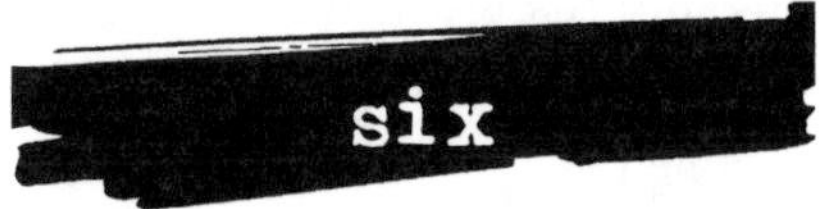

The Respiratory System

The job of the respiratory system is to bring oxygen into the body and remove carbon dioxide. Oxygen is essential for the cells of our bodies to produce energy; carbon dioxide is a waste product from the cells. The main components of the respiratory system are the lungs and airways, which include the nose, mouth, larynx, trachea, and bronchial tubes. Caused by bacteria, viruses, and pollutants in the air, respiratory illnesses can reduce the amount of oxygen taken into the body.

Asthma

Asthma is a chronic inflammation that constricts the airways in the lungs. It can cause shortness of breath, tightness in the chest, coughing, and wheezing. Triggers that worsen these symptoms include air pollution, infection, pollen, overexertion, certain foods, tobacco smoke, cold air, and chemical and factory fumes.

❁ Anise and Chamomile Vapors

1½ teaspoons aniseeds, crushed
1 teaspoon dried chamomile, crumbled
1 cup water, boiled

Lightly toast the aniseeds in a dry frying pan over low heat, and then crush. Pre-warm a cup or mug with hot tap water before adding the aniseeds, chamomile, and boiled water. Cover and steep for 15 to 20 minutes, and then strain.

To use: Warm the tea to the point where it is steaming. Hold the mug near your face to inhale the vapors. Drink the tea when it is comfortably warm.

❁ Hyssop and Spearmint Tea

1 teaspoon dried hyssop, crumbled
1 teaspoon dried spearmint, crumbled
1 cup water, boiled

Pre-warm a cup or mug with hot tap water, and then add the hyssop, spearmint, and boiled water. Cover and steep for 10 to 15 minutes before straining.

To use: Warm the tea slightly and add honey to taste. Drink a cup as needed.

Chamomile is a gentle antihistamine that can help prevent asthma attacks. However, while it is an antiallergenic for most people, those who have allergies to plants in the Asteraceae/Compositae (aster/daisy) family should check for sensitivity before using chamomile. Hyssop helps relieve the heavy feeling in the chest. A steam inhalation can also be used for asthma, but keep the bath towel tent open so the steam is not overwhelming. Other herbs that help ease asthma include bay laurel, black cohosh, dill, fennel, ginger, lemon balm, mullein, nettle, oregano, parsley, peppermint, rosemary, sage, thyme, and turmeric.

Bronchitis

Bronchitis is an infection or irritation of the bronchial tubes, which are the large passageways that carry air in and out of the lungs. Bronchitis often develops from a cold or other respiratory infection and more commonly occurs during the winter. Symptoms can include persistent coughing, thick phlegm, discomfort in the chest, wheezing, shortness of breath, fatigue, and a slight fever.

❁ Hyssop and Peppermint Tea

1½ teaspoons dried hyssop, crumbled
½ teaspoon dried peppermint, crumbled
1 cup water, boiled

Pre-warm a mug or cup with hot tap water, and then add the hyssop, peppermint, and boiled water. Cover and steep for 15 to 20 minutes before straining.

> ***To use:*** Warm slightly and add honey to taste. Drink 2 to 4 cups a day.

❁ Rosemary and Fennel Tincture

½ cup dried rosemary, crumbled
¼ cup fennel seeds, crushed

2 cups 80 to 100 proof alcohol (vodka, gin, brandy, or rum)

Before crushing, lightly toast the fennel seeds in a dry frying pan over low heat. Combine the fennel seeds, rosemary, and alcohol in a glass jar with a tight-fitting lid. Close and shake for 1 to 2 minutes. Set aside for 2 to 4 weeks, shaking the jar every other day. Strain and store in a dark glass bottle.

To use: Dilute 1 teaspoon in a cup of water, tea, or fruit juice. Take up to 3 times a day.

Hyssop is a powerful herb with anti-inflammatory and antibacterial properties, making it effective for a range of respiratory problems. As an expectorant, it helps clear and cleanse the lungs and fight infection. It also relieves bronchial spasms. Combining hyssop with peppermint provides the added benefit of menthol. The anti-inflammatory and antispasmodic properties of rosemary and fennel make the tincture especially helpful for chronic bronchitis. The Fennel and Coriander Tea included under Cough works well, too. Steam inhalation relieves coughing and helps open the airways. Other herbs that can be used for bronchitis include angelica, anise, basil, black cohosh, caraway, dill, garlic, lemon balm, mullein, oregano, spearmint, and thyme.

Catarrh

Catarrh is the excessive buildup and discharge of mucus in the nose, sinuses, and throat. Accompanied by inflammation of the mucous membranes, it is usually caused by a cold, hay fever, or other type of allergy.

❁ Oregano and Mullein Steam Inhalation

4 tablespoons dried oregano, crumbled
3 tablespoons dried mullein, crumbled
1 quart water

Place the oregano, mullein, and water in a saucepan and bring to a boil. Cover and simmer on low heat for 1 to 2 minutes. Remove the saucepan from the stove.

> ***To use:*** Place a bath towel over your head to create a tent above the steaming water. Close your eyes and hold your face a comfortable distance from the water so the steam will not be too hot. Stay under the tent for 3 to 5 minutes or until the water is no longer steaming.

❁ Hyssop Infusion

5 tablespoons dried hyssop, crumbled
1 quart water, boiled

Warm a large glass jar with hot tap water, and then add the hyssop and boiled water. Cover and steep for 35 to 45 minutes before straining. Store in the refrigerator.

> ***To use:*** Drink a cup at a time, warming and adding honey or lemon to taste. Take 1 to 3 cups a day.

The warm steam of mullein and oregano soothes irritation and disinfects the inflamed mucous membranes. Hyssop is an excellent expectorant and is especially helpful when dealing with chronic catarrh. Other herbs to use include garlic, sage, St. John's wort, and thyme.

Common Cold

The common cold is an upper respiratory infection that can be caused by a variety of viruses. It usually goes away within two weeks. Symptoms can include a runny or stuffy nose, chest congestion, cough, sore throat, watery eyes, sneezing, and headache. A low-grade fever and muscle aches may also occur. With many symptoms in common, it is often difficult to tell the difference between a common cold and the flu.

❁ Lemon Balm and Peppermint Infusion

4 tablespoons dried lemon balm, crumbled
2 tablespoons dried peppermint, crumbled
1 quart water, boiled

Pre-warm a large glass jar with hot tap water before adding the lemon balm, peppermint, and boiled water. Cover and steep for 30 to 40 minutes, and then strain. Store in the refrigerator.

To use: Warm and drink a cup at a time. Take 3 to 4 cups a day.

❁ Ginger and Bay Steam Inhalation

3 tablespoons fresh ginger, coarsely grated
3 tablespoons dried bay laurel, crumbled
1 quart water

Place the water and ginger in a saucepan, cover, and bring to boil. Reduce the heat and simmer for 4 or 5 minutes before stirring in the bay laurel. Simmer for another 1 or 2 minutes, and then remove the saucepan from the stove.

> ***To use:*** Place a bath towel over your head to create a tent above the steaming water. Close your eyes and hold your face a comfortable distance from the water so the steam will not be too hot. Stay under the tent for 3 to 5 minutes or until the water is no longer steaming.

The antiviral components in lemon balm make it ideal to ease the symptoms of colds and flu; its antioxidants support and strengthen the immune system. In addition to bringing soothing relief, the nutrients in peppermint aid recovery from illness. While bay laurel and ginger have antiviral and expectorant properties, ginger is also an anti-inflammatory that helps soothe and clear the airways.

Sage can help prevent colds by simply using it in food, but if illness strikes, sage tea eases cold and flu symptoms. Eating garlic during a cold can help reduce symptoms, and by keeping it in your diet, it can help prevent a recurrence. Fresh, raw garlic works best. Add a sliced clove to a salad and keep aniseeds handy for your breath. Other herbs to use when dealing with a cold include angelica, anise, basil, burdock, cayenne, chamomile, dill, hyssop, lavender, mullein, oregano, rosemary, spearmint, thyme, and yarrow.

Congestion

The most common causes of chest and nasal congestion are the common cold or flu; however, it can also result from allergies, sinusitis, and other more serious infections. Excess mucus is the major symptom but sneezing and coughing are also common.

❁ Cayenne Tea

1 pinch cayenne, powdered
1 teaspoon lemon juice
1 teaspoon honey
1 cup water, boiled

Pre-warm a cup or mug with hot tap water before adding the cayenne, lemon juice, and boiled water. Stir in a spoonful of honey.

To use: Allow the tea to cool just enough to drink. Take 1 or 2 cups a day.

❁ Thyme, Rosemary, and Peppermint Steam Inhalation

3 tablespoons dried thyme, crumbled
2 tablespoons dried rosemary, crumbled
1 tablespoon dried peppermint, crumbled
1 quart water

Place the water, thyme, rosemary, and peppermint in a saucepan, cover, and bring to a boil. Reduce the heat and simmer for 1 or 2 minutes. Remove the saucepan from the stove.

To use: Place a bath towel over your head to create a tent above the steaming water. Close your eyes and hold your face a comfortable distance from the water so the steam will not be too hot. Stay under the tent for 3 to 5 minutes or until the water is no longer steaming.

Also try an infusion of oregano, thyme, and sage in equal amounts to drink or to make a warm compress for the chest. A steam inhalation with bay laurel also helps clear the airways. Other herbs that help relieve congestion include angelica, anise, caraway, dill, fennel, garlic, ginger, hyssop, lemon balm, mullein, spearmint, and St. John's wort.

Cough

Coughing is the body's way of removing bacteria, mucus, and other irritants from the throat and lungs. Colds and the flu are the most common causes of a cough, but it can also occur as a result of allergies, postnasal drip, gastroesophageal reflux disease (GERD), and other conditions.

❁ Anise and Lemon Balm Syrup

4 tablespoons aniseeds, crushed
4 tablespoons dried lemon balm, crumbled
1 quart water
1 cup honey

Before crushing, lightly toast the aniseeds in a dry frying pan over low heat. Combine the aniseeds, lemon balm, and water in a saucepan, cover, and bring to a boil. Reduce the heat to as low as possible and simmer at least 30 minutes or until the volume is reduced by half. Strain out the herbs, return 2 cups of liquid to the saucepan, and add the honey. Warm on low heat, stirring until the mixture is smooth. Remove from the heat, allow the mixture to cool slightly, and then pour into a glass jar with a tight-fitting lid. Store in the refrigerator where it will keep for several weeks.

To use: Take 1 teaspoon as needed.

❁ Fennel and Coriander Tea

1½ teaspoons fennel seeds, crushed
½ teaspoon coriander seeds, crushed
1 cup water, boiled

Lightly toast the fennel and coriander seeds in a dry frying pan over low heat before crushing. Pre-warm a cup or mug with hot tap water, and then add the seeds and boiled water. Cover and steep for 15 minutes before straining.

To use: Warm slightly before drinking. Take 2 to 3 cups a day.

Spicy-sweet and licorice-like, anise may be a familiar taste in commercial cough syrups and lozenges, but it does more than add flavor. A tea made with the seeds or a strong infusion of the leaves eases coughs and acts as an expectorant. Hyssop and thyme also combine well for a cough syrup. The antispasmodic properties of fennel and coriander are especially good for chronic coughs; fennel is also an expectorant. Other herbs to use include angelica, basil, black cohosh, caraway, dill, garlic, ginger, lemongrass, mullein, oregano, parsley, peppermint, and spearmint.

Flu

Influenza, more commonly known as the flu, is a viral infection. As mentioned, it is frequently difficult to distinguish from a cold; however, the flu is often more severe and can lead to complications and even death. Flu symptoms can include headache, aches and pains in joints and muscles, pain around the eyes, weakness and fatigue, chest congestion, cough, a runny or stuffy nose, sore throat, and fever. The elderly, young children, and people with certain medical conditions are at a higher risk of developing serious complications.

❁ Rosemary, Sage, and Thyme Chest Rub

For the infused oil:
1 tablespoon dried rosemary, crumbled
1 tablespoon dried sage, crumbled
1 tablespoon dried thyme, crumbled
⅔ cup coconut oil

For the chest rub:
½ ounce beeswax, chopped into small pieces
8–9 tablespoons infused oil

Combine the rosemary, sage, thyme, and coconut oil in a double boiler and cover. With the heat as low as possible, warm for 40 minutes. Remove from the heat and allow it to cool slightly before straining. Combine the infused oil and beeswax in a glass jar in a saucepan of water. Warm over low heat, stirring until the beeswax melts. Remove from the heat and allow the mixture to cool slightly. Test the consistency and adjust if necessary. Allow it to cool completely before using or storing.

To use: Rub a little on the chest as needed, especially overnight.

❁ Bay and Lavender Bath Infusion

1½ cups dried bay laurel, crumbled
1½ cups dried lavender, crumbled
4–5 quarts water

Place the bay laurel and lavender in a muslin bag and set aside. Bring the water to a boil in a large stockpot, and then turn off the heat. Add the herb bag to the water, cover, and steep for 2 hours.

To use: Warm to a comfortable temperature, and then add the infusion and bag of herbs to bathwater.

In addition to easing flu symptoms, the antiviral properties of rosemary, sage, and thyme fight infection while providing support for the immune system. The Bay and Lavender Bath Infusion provides a cleansing soak with vapors that help relieve congestion and headache. A steam inhalation with lemon balm and peppermint can relieve congestion, sinus pressure, and headache. Herbal tea taken three or four times a day also helps soothe symptoms and recover from the flu. Other herbs that help relieve symptoms include anise, basil, cayenne, garlic, ginger, hyssop, mullein, oregano, and yarrow.

Hay Fever

Allergic rhinitis, more commonly known as hay fever, is a seasonal allergy caused by the immune system's overreaction to an outdoor allergen such as grass, mold, and pollen. When an allergen is detected, special cells release a chemical called *histamine* into the blood stream to activate the body's defenses. The major symptoms of hay fever are respiratory congestion, itchy and/or watery eyes, and a runny nose.

❁ Parsley Infusion

5 tablespoons dried parsley, crumbled
1 quart water, boiled

Pre-warm a large glass jar with hot tap water, and then add the parsley and boiled water. Cover and steep for 45 minutes before straining. Store in the refrigerator.

> ***To use:*** Warm and drink a cup at a time. Take 2 to 4 cups a day.

❁ Nettle and St. John's Wort Syrup

4 tablespoons dried nettle, crumbled
4 tablespoons dried St. John's wort, crumbled
1 quart water
1 cup honey

Combine the nettle, St. John's wort, and water in a saucepan, cover, and bring to a boil. Reduce the heat to as low as possible and simmer at least 30 minutes or until the volume is reduced by half. Strain out the herbs, return 2 cups of liquid to the saucepan, and add the honey. Warm over low heat, stirring until the mixture is smooth. Remove from the heat, allow the mixture to cool slightly, and then pour into a glass jar with a tight-fitting lid. Store in the refrigerator where it will keep for several weeks.

To use: Take 2 teaspoons straight, 2 or 3 times a day.

The parsley infusion can also be used to make a warm compress to relieve puffy eyes. Ginger also reduces allergic inflammation. Although chamomile is an antiallergenic for most people, those who have allergies to plants in the Asteraceae/Compositae (aster/daisy) family should check for sensitivity before using it. Thyme can also ease hay fever.

There is no scientific evidence to support the popular belief that using local honey eases hay fever symptoms. What does help is keeping carpets and upholstered furniture clean, using an air purifier, and placing allergen-proof covers on bed pillows.

Laryngitis

Laryngitis is the inflammation of the larynx, also known as the voice box. Inflammation can be caused by irritation, overuse, and infection. Laryngitis often occurs with allergies, asthma, the common cold, and the flu. Symptoms include a scratchy, husky, or weak voice. The best treatment is to rest the voice.

❁ Spearmint and St. John's Wort Honey

¼ cup dried spearmint, crumbled
¼ cup dried St. John's wort, crumbled
1 cup honey

Place the spearmint and St. John's wort in a small muslin bag in a glass jar and add the honey. Set the jar in a saucepan of water and warm over low heat for 30 minutes. Remove from the heat and set aside overnight.

To use: Place a teaspoon in tea or take it straight. Take 2 to 3 times a day.

❁ Lavender and Peppermint Spray

6 tablespoons dried lavender, crumbled
5 tablespoons dried peppermint, crumbled
1 quart water, boiled

Pre-warm a large glass jar with hot tap water, and then add the lavender, peppermint, and boiled water. Cover and steep for 1 hour before straining. Allow it to cool completely before using or storing.

To use: Pour into a spray bottle with a fine mister. Use as a throat spray as needed.

An herbal steam inhalation also helps soothe the throat. Other herbs to use for laryngitis include chamomile, fennel, hyssop, mullein, sage, thyme, and yarrow.

Sinusitis

Sinusitis is an infection of the sinuses caused by bacteria or a virus. Symptoms can include nasal congestion, facial pain, frontal headache, fever, and chills. Sinusitis often occurs with the common cold but can also be caused by allergies, swelling of the nasal tissue, and nasal polyps.

❁ Lemon Balm and Basil Steam Inhalation

4 tablespoons dried lemon balm, crumbled
3 tablespoons dried basil, crumbled
1 quart water

Place the water, lemon balm, and basil in a saucepan and bring to a boil. Cover and simmer on low heat for 1 or 2 minutes. Remove the saucepan from the stove.

> ***To use:*** Place a bath towel over your head to create a tent above the steaming water. Close your eyes and hold your face a comfortable distance from the water so the steam will not be too hot. Stay under the tent for 3 to 5 minutes or until the water is no longer steaming.

❁ Garlic Syrup

3–4 garlic cloves, crushed
½ cup honey

Place the garlic cloves in a small muslin bag and crush them. Place the bag and honey in a jar and let it stand for 2 to 3 hours. Stir and remove the bag of garlic.

> ***To use:*** Take 1 teaspoon 2 to 3 times a day.

A warm steam inhalation with infection-fighting herbs eases swollen nasal passages and soothes irritation. The antiviral and antibacterial properties of garlic make it an excellent choice for treating sinusitis. The compounds that are excreted through the lungs and cause garlic breath put the healing components of this herb right where they are needed for respiratory illnesses. Cooked garlic is effective but raw cloves are more potent. You may want to keep aniseeds or parsley leaves on hand for your breath. Other herbs to use for sinusitis include angelica, anise, bay laurel, ginger, hyssop, lavender, peppermint, rosemary, sage, St. John's wort, and thyme. A saline nasal spray also helps.

Sore Throat

Usually caused by viral infections, most sore throats last only a few days. They generally accompany the common cold and flu. A sore throat is often the first sign of illness. Symptoms include scratchiness or irritation that feels worse when swallowing.

❁ Lavender and Sage Gargle

1 teaspoon dried lavender, crumbled
1 teaspoon dried sage, crumbled
½ teaspoon table salt
1 cup water, boiled

Pre-warm a cup or mug with hot tap water before adding the lavender, sage, salt, and boiled water. Cover and steep for 15 minutes, and then strain.

To use: Warm to a comfortable temperature, and then gargle with a little at a time until it is gone. Gargle 2 or 3 times a day or as needed.

❁ Peppermint and Burdock Tea

1½ teaspoons dried peppermint, crumbled
½ teaspoon dried burdock, crumbled
1 cup water, boiled

Pre-warm a cup or mug with hot tap water before adding the peppermint, burdock, and boiled water. Cover and steep for 15 minutes, and then strain.

> ***To use:*** Warm to a comfortable temperature, adding a teaspoon of honey to taste. Drink slowly so the heat can soothe your throat.

The anti-inflammatory and antiseptic properties of burdock, lavender, peppermint, and sage help relieve and heal a sore throat. A teaspoon of tincture in a cup of warm water can be used as a gargle, too. Other herbs that help relieve a sore throat include bay laurel, black cohosh, cayenne, chamomile, fennel, garlic, ginger, hyssop, lemongrass, mullein, oregano, rosemary, spearmint, thyme, and yarrow.

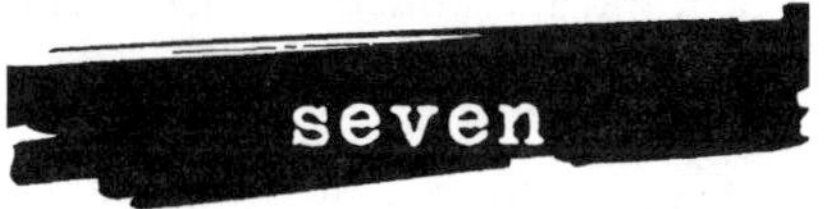

The Digestive System

The digestive system consists of a series of organs that convert food into nutrients that the body can absorb. It is also responsible for processing nondigestible waste and elimination. Some herbs can be used for a range of digestive issues, which is fortunate as many ailments do not occur in isolation.

Belching

A belch or burp is caused by the release of excess air from the stomach, which can ease minor digestive discomfort. Some of the causes for swallowing excess air include eating or drinking too quickly, chewing gum, and drinking carbonated beverages. Chronic belching can be caused by gastritis (inflammation of the stomach lining) and heartburn.

❁ Chamomile and Spearmint Tea

1 teaspoon dried chamomile, crumbled
1 teaspoon dried spearmint, crumbled
1 cup water, boiled

Pre-warm a cup or mug with hot tap water before adding the chamomile, spearmint, and boiled water. Cover and steep for 10 minutes, and then strain.

To use: Drink a cup after meals when discomfort occurs.

❁ Caraway and Fennel Tea

1½ teaspoons caraway seeds, crushed
½ teaspoon fennel seeds, crushed
1 cup water, boiled

Lightly toast the caraway and fennel seeds in a dry frying pan over low heat before crushing. Pre-warm a cup or mug with hot tap water, and then add the seeds and boiled water. Cover and steep for 15 to 20 minutes before straining.

To use: Drink a cup after meals when discomfort occurs.

Adding a few mint leaves to water that you drink with a meal or afterward also helps, as does chewing a few caraway seeds. Peppermint and ginger are also effective to ease belching.

Bloating

Bloating occurs when excess air is not passed by belching or flatulence and instead builds up in the stomach or intestines. It can be accompanied by abdominal pain and/or feeling uncomfortably full. Some of the causes for bloating include eating fatty foods, eating too quickly, stress or anxiety, and lactose intolerance.

❁ Thyme Honey

½ cup dried thyme, crumbled
1 cup honey

Place the thyme in a small muslin bag. Pour the honey into a slightly larger jar and set it in a saucepan of water. Warm over low heat until the honey becomes a little less viscous, and then add the bag of thyme. Use a butter knife to submerge it in the honey. Continue warming for 15 to 20 minutes. Remove from the heat and set aside until it cools. Store in a cupboard at room temperature for a week. To remove the bag of thyme, heat the jar in a saucepan of water over low heat. Squeeze excess honey from the bag.

To use: Add a teaspoon to a cup of tea, or take it straight as needed.

❁ Coriander and Dandelion Tincture

½ cup coriander seeds, crushed
¼ cup dried dandelion leaves, crumbled
2 cups 80 to 100 proof alcohol (vodka, gin, brandy, or rum)

Before crushing, lightly toast the coriander seeds in a dry frying pan over low heat. Place the coriander seeds, dandelion, and alcohol in a glass jar with a tight-fitting lid. Close and shake for 1 to 2 minutes. Set aside for 2 to 3 weeks, shaking the jar every other day. Strain and store in a dark glass bottle.

> ***To use:*** Take ½ teaspoon straight or in a cup of water, tea, or fruit juice. Take up to 3 times a day.

An herbal tea after meals or as needed is also effective to ease bloating. Cooking with any of the herbs mentioned here can help, too. Other herbs that reduce bloating include angelica, anise, bay laurel, caraway, chamomile, fennel, ginger, hyssop, lavender, peppermint, and rosemary.

Colic

Crying and fussing are normal behaviors for a newborn baby. However, when episodes are intense and have no apparent reason, colic may be the issue, especially if episodes last for several hours three or more days a week. Colic is a pain in the abdomen that is usually caused by intestinal gas or sometimes an obstruction. It occurs most often in the evening and may be accompanied by your baby arching their back and tensing the body.

❁ Chamomile Tea

1 teaspoon dried chamomile, crumbled
1 cup water, boiled

After pre-warming a cup or mug with hot tap water, add the chamomile and boiled water. Cover and steep for 15 minutes before straining.

> ***To use:*** With a medicine dropper, give your baby a teaspoon or two at a time.

In addition to tea, give your baby a warm bath or gently rub their belly. Spearmint can also relieve colic. When taken as tea by the mother, caraway, dill, and fennel help increase the supply of breast milk and relieve a baby's colic. If crying and other symptoms are excessive, schedule a visit with your baby's doctor.

Constipation

Although the frequency of bowel movements varies from person to person, constipation is generally defined as having three or fewer a week. Some of the causes include lack of exercise, eating too much junk food, alcohol, caffeine, lack of fiber in the diet, and an insufficient amount of water. A change in routine, especially when traveling, can also cause constipation.

❁ Burdock and Ginger Decoction

4 tablespoons fresh burdock root, chopped
2 tablespoons fresh ginger, chopped
1 quart water

Place the burdock, ginger, and water in a saucepan and bring to a boil. Stir, cover, and reduce the heat to as low as possible. Gently simmer for 30 minutes, and then allow it to cool completely before straining. Store in the refrigerator.

To use: Warm and drink a cup at a time. Take 2 to 4 cups a day.

❁ Parsley and Dandelion Tea

2 teaspoons fresh parsley, chopped
2 teaspoons fresh dandelion leaves, chopped
1 cup water, boiled

Pre-warm a cup or mug with hot tap water before adding the parsley, dandelion, and boiled water. Cover and steep for 15 minutes, and then strain.

To use: Drink a cup after meals and before bed.

Burdock, ginger, and dandelion are especially good for encouraging peristalsis (the motion of the muscles in the digestive tract) to help get things moving. Exercise also helps. Other herbs that ease constipation include basil, dill, and oregano. Be sure to drink at least eight to ten glasses of water a day. If you add or increase fiber in your diet, do so gradually to avoid bloating and gas.

Diarrhea

Everyone occasionally experiences diarrhea: loose, watery, and sometimes more frequent bowel movements. It is often accompanied by abdominal cramps and bloating. Common causes include contaminated food or water, viruses, lactose intolerance, fructose, artificial sweeteners, medications, and digestive disorders.

❁ Peppermint and Thyme Tincture

¾ cup fresh peppermint, chopped
¾ cup fresh thyme, chopped

2 cups 80 to 100 proof alcohol (vodka, gin, brandy, or rum)

Place the peppermint, thyme, and alcohol in a jar with a tight-fitting lid. Close and shake for 1 to 2 minutes. Set aside for 3 weeks, shaking the jar every other day. Strain and store in a dark glass bottle.

To use: Take 1 teaspoon diluted in an ounce of water 2 or 3 times a day. It can also be taken straight by putting 10 to 15 drops under the tongue.

❁ Sage Tea

1–1½ teaspoons dried sage, crumbled
1 cup water, boiled

Pre-warm a cup or mug with hot tap water, and then add the sage and boiled water. Cover and steep for 15 minutes before straining.

To use: Drink up to 3 cups a day, but not for more than 3 days.

The Peppermint and Thyme Tincture can be used for other digestive problems, such as flatulence and indigestion. Cayenne, coriander, and mullein can be used to ease diarrhea, too. While coping with diarrhea, it helps to stay hydrated and to eat food that is easy to digest such as rice, cooked potatoes, bananas, and applesauce.

Flatulence

Flatulence is the passing of intestinal gas through the anus. Some of the causes include swallowed air that is not released through burping, the breakdown of undigested food, and lactose intolerance. Flatulence can be accompanied by bloating and belly or side pain.

❁ Angelica and Burdock Decoction

4 tablespoons dried angelica root, chopped
2 tablespoons dried burdock root, chopped
1 quart water

Place the angelica, burdock, and water in a saucepan and bring to a boil. Stir, cover, and reduce the heat to as low as possible. Gently simmer for 20 to 25 minutes, and then allow it to cool completely before straining. Store in the refrigerator.

To use: Warm and drink a cup at a time. Take 2 times a day or as needed.

❁ Oregano and Lemongrass Tea

1 teaspoon dried oregano, crumbled
1 teaspoon dried lemongrass, crumbled
1 cup water, boiled

Pre-warm a cup or mug with hot tap water before adding the oregano, lemongrass, and boiled water. Cover and steep for 10 minutes, and then strain.

To use: Drink a cup after meals or whenever you feel gassy.

Chewing a few caraway seeds after meals can also reduce flatulence. Other herbs to use for this issue include anise, basil, bay laurel, cayenne, chamomile, coriander, dill, fennel, ginger, hyssop, lavender, lemon balm, parsley, peppermint, rosemary, spearmint, thyme, and turmeric.

Heartburn/GERD

Commonly known as heartburn and acid indigestion, gastroesophageal reflux disease (GERD) is a disorder of the lower esophageal sphincter muscle located between the bottom of the esophagus and the stomach. Heartburn is characterized by a burning sensation in the chest. Some of the causes for heartburn include overeating, eating just before bedtime, certain foods or drinks, stress, alcohol, smoking, and hiatal hernia.

❁ Dill Water

4 teaspoons dillseeds
2 pinches salt
1 quart water

Place the seeds and salt in a jar with just enough water to cover them. Soak for 7 hours, and then drain off the water. Place 1 quart of fresh water in a saucepan, add the seeds, and bring to a boil. Reduce the heat and gently simmer for 10 minutes. Cool completely before straining. Store in the refrigerator for up to 2 days.

To use: Drink ½ cup at a time, up to 2 or 3 cups a day.

❁ Ginger and Coriander Decoction

4 tablespoons fresh ginger, chopped
3 tablespoons coriander seeds, crushed
1 quart water

Lightly toast the coriander seeds in a dry frying pan before crushing. Combine the coriander seeds, ginger, and water in a saucepan and bring to a boil. Stir, cover, and reduce the heat to as low as possible. Gently simmer for 30 minutes, and then allow it to cool completely before straining. Store in the refrigerator.

To use: Warm and drink a cup at a time. Take 2 or 3 times a day or as needed.

With its antispasmodic properties, chamomile tea helps relieve heartburn and is especially good to take before bedtime as it aids restful sleep. Chamomile also helps heal damage to the esophagus. A tincture made with any of the herbs mentioned here also works well; take ½ to 1 teaspoon in warm water two or three times a day. Although peppermint can ease heartburn, it does not work for everyone and can occasionally aggravate the discomfort. Other herbs to use for heartburn include angelica, caraway, fennel, lemon balm, and spearmint. In a pinch, if you have a jar of dill pickles, drink some of the juice for relief.

Hemorrhoids

Also known as piles, hemorrhoids are swollen veins in and around the anus. Similar to varicose veins in the legs, the blood vessels become stretched due to pressure. Some of the causes for hemorrhoids include straining during bowel movements, pressure on the bowels during pregnancy, prolonged sitting, and heavy lifting. Symptoms can include discomfort, pain, irritation, burning, and itching.

❁ Yarrow and Lavender Gel

For the infused oil:
1 tablespoon dried yarrow, crumbled
1 tablespoon dried lavender, crumbled
½ cup coconut oil

For the gel:
6–8 tablespoons aloe vera gel
½ cup infused oil

Place the yarrow, lavender, and coconut oil in a double boiler and cover. With the heat as low as possible, warm for 30 minutes. Remove from the heat, allow the infused oil to cool completely, and then strain. Place the aloe vera gel in a bowl and slowly add the infused oil until the gel reaches a consistency you like. Gently stir until it is thoroughly mixed. Store in a glass jar with a tight-fitting lid.

To use: Apply several times a day or as needed.

❁ Cilantro and Dill Salve

For the infused oil:
4 teaspoons fresh cilantro (coriander) leaves, chopped
4 teaspoons fresh dill, chopped
½ cup coconut oil

For the salve:
½ ounce beeswax, chopped into small pieces
7–8 tablespoons infused oil

Place the cilantro, dill, and coconut oil in a double boiler and cover. With the heat as low as possible, warm for 30 minutes. Remove from the heat and allow the infused oil to cool slightly before straining. Place the beeswax and infused oil in a glass jar and set it in a saucepan of water. Warm over low heat, stirring until the beeswax melts. Remove from the heat and allow the mixture to cool completely before using or storing.

To use: Apply several times a day or as needed.

All the ingredients in the gel and salve recipes have anti-inflammatory properties; yarrow and cilantro are also astringent, which aids in shrinking hemorrhoids. Other treatments include the application of plain witch hazel and a strong herbal infusion for a sitz bath. Chamomile, dandelion, mullein, nettle, sage, and St. John's wort can also be used to ease hemorrhoids.

Indigestion

Dyspepsia, commonly known as indigestion or upset stomach, is discomfort or pain in the upper abdomen that can be caused by overeating, eating spicy or greasy foods, lack of exercise, and hiatal hernia. Other symptoms include belching, bloating, flatulence, nausea, and heartburn. Consult your doctor if you have chronic indigestion.

❁ Oregano, Anise, and Lemon Balm Tea

1 teaspoon dried oregano, crumbled
½ teaspoon aniseeds, crushed
½ teaspoon dried lemon balm, crumbled
1 cup water, boiled

Before crushing the aniseeds, lightly toast them in a dry frying pan over low heat. Pre-warm a cup or mug with hot tap water, and then add the oregano, lemon balm, aniseeds, and boiled water. Cover and steep for 10 to 15 minutes before straining.

> ***To use:*** Drink a cup as needed. Take up to 2 or 3 cups a day.

❁ Fennel and Turmeric Tincture

½ cup fennel seeds, crushed
¼ cup dried turmeric, chopped
2 cups 80 to 100 proof alcohol (vodka, gin, brandy, or rum)

Before crushing, lightly toast the fennel seeds in a dry frying pan over low heat. Combine the fennel seeds, turmeric, and alcohol in a glass jar with a tight-fitting lid. Close and shake for 1 to 2 minutes. Set aside for 2 to 3 weeks, shaking the jar every other day. Strain and store in a dark glass bottle.

> ***To use:*** Take ½ to 1 teaspoon when indigestion strikes. Alternatively, add 1 teaspoon of the tincture to a cup of boiled water for tea.

A cup of dandelion root decoction works well as does munching on a few caraway seeds. The Dill Water included under Heartburn/GERD also eases indigestion. Other herbs that can be used include angelica, basil, bay laurel, chamomile, coriander, ginger, hyssop, lavender, lemongrass, mullein, peppermint, rosemary, spearmint, thyme, valerian, and yarrow.

Irritable Bowel Syndrome (IBS)

IBS is a disorder that affects the large intestine and impairs the movement of food and waste. Some of the symptoms include abdominal cramping or pain, nausea, bloating, excess gas, diarrhea, and constipation. The cause of IBS is unknown.

❁ Caraway and Peppermint Infusion

2½ tablespoons caraway seeds, crushed
1 tablespoon dried peppermint, crumbled
1 quart water, boiled

Lightly toast the caraway seeds in a dry frying pan over low heat before crushing. Pre-warm a large glass jar with hot tap water, and then add the seeds, peppermint, and boiled water. Cover and steep for 35 to 40 minutes before straining. Store in the refrigerator.

> ***To use:*** Warm a cup at a time and drink up to 2 or 3 cups a day.

❁ Angelica Decoction

5 tablespoons dried angelica root, chopped
1 quart water

Place the angelica and water in a saucepan and bring to a boil. Stir, cover, and reduce the heat to as low as possible. Simmer for 25 minutes, and then allow it to cool completely before straining. Store in the refrigerator.

> ***To use:*** Warm and drink a cup at a time between meals. Drink up to 3 cups a day.

The anti-inflammatory and antispasmodic properties of angelica, caraway, and peppermint ease abdominal pain and other symptoms. Peppermint also aids in balancing intestinal flora. Chamomile, fennel, lemon balm, rosemary, and garlic also help when dealing with IBS. However, garlic does not work for everyone and should be experimented with carefully. Because IBS varies widely from person to person, it helps keep a food diary to determine specific triggers.

Nausea

Nausea is the unpleasant, queasy feeling in the stomach that often occurs just before vomiting. It may be accompanied by sweating, increased salivation, and trembling. Some of the causes include stomach virus, migraine, middle ear infection, stress, and food poisoning.

❁ Chamomile and Spearmint Tea

1 teaspoon dried chamomile, crumbled
1 teaspoon dried spearmint, crumbled
1 cup water, boiled

Pre-warm a cup or mug with hot tap water before adding the chamomile, spearmint, and boiled water. Cover and steep for 10 to 15 minutes, and then strain.

To use: Drink a little at a time as needed.

❁ Coriander and Anise Tea

½ teaspoon coriander seeds, crushed
½ teaspoon aniseeds, crushed
1 cup water, boiled

Before crushing the coriander and aniseeds, lightly toast them in a dry frying pan over low heat. Pre-warm a cup or mug with hot tap water, and then add the seeds and boiled water. Cover and steep for 10 to 15 minutes before straining.

To use: Sip a little at a time as needed.

For mild nausea, add a few peppermint leaves to a glass of water or lemonade. Other herbs that ease nausea include basil, fennel, ginger, and turmeric.

Stomach Pain

Stomach pain can range from mild to sharp pain or cramp in the stomach or abdomen. Some common causes include indigestion, constipation, stomach virus, food allergies, gas, food poisoning, lactose intolerance, and irritable bowel syndrome.

❁ Lemongrass and Hyssop Tea

1½ teaspoons dried lemongrass, crumbled
½ teaspoon dried hyssop, crumbled
1 cup water, boiled

Pre-warm a cup or mug with hot tap water, and then add the lemongrass, hyssop, and boiled water. Cover and steep for 10 to 15 minutes before straining.

To use: Warm before drinking. Take 1 to 2 cups a day.

❁ Basil and Yarrow Tincture

½ cup dried basil, crumbled
¼ cup dried yarrow, crumbled
2 cups 80 to 100 proof alcohol (vodka, gin, brandy, or rum)

Place the basil, yarrow, and alcohol in a glass jar with a tight-fitting lid. Close and shake for 1 to 2 minutes. Set aside for 2 to 4 weeks, shaking the jar every other day. Strain and store in a dark glass bottle.

To use: Pre-warm a cup or mug, and then add 1 teaspoon of the tincture and a cup of boiled water. Drink twice a day.

The anti-inflammatory and antispasmodic properties of lemongrass and hyssop ease stomach pain. They also help with flatulence and indigestion, which may be related to the stomach pain. In addition to easing pain, basil and yarrow support healthy digestion. The sweet but savory taste of basil balances the bitterness of yarrow. Other herbs to use for stomach pain include angelica, anise, caraway, cayenne, chamomile, coriander, dill, fennel, lemon balm, peppermint, rosemary, thyme, turmeric, and valerian.

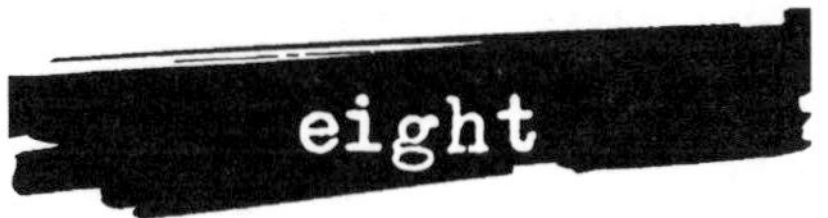

The Integumentary System (Skin)

The skin is the largest sensory organ of the body and the major component of the integumentary system. It acts as a protective barrier that provides the body's first line of defense against disease and pollution. The skin also helps regulate body temperature and maintain a balance of fluids. In addition to the skin, the integumentary system includes hair, nails, and the exocrine glands (sweat glands and tear ducts).

Acne

This common skin problem usually occurs when hair follicles become plugged with oil and dead skin cells. Acne can also be caused by excess oil production and bacteria. It is often aggravated by hormonal changes, diet, some medications, and stress. Although acne is most common among teenagers, it can affect people of all ages.

❁ **Rosemary, Lemon Balm, Lavender, and Chamomile Vinegar**

3 teaspoons dried rosemary, crumbled

2 teaspoons dried lemon balm, crumbled
2 teaspoons dried lavender, crumbled
2 teaspoons dried chamomile, crumbled
¼–½ cup vinegar

Place the rosemary, lemon balm, lavender, chamomile, and vinegar in a glass jar with a tight-fitting lid. Add a little more vinegar if necessary to cover the plant material. Steep for at least 2 weeks before straining.

> ***To use:*** After washing your face, gently dab the mixture onto the affected areas with a cotton swab or cotton ball.

❁ Burdock and Dandelion Decoction

1½ tablespoons dried burdock root, chopped
1½ tablespoons dried dandelion root, chopped
2 cups water

Place the burdock, dandelion, and water in a saucepan and bring to a boil. Stir, cover, and reduce the heat to as low as possible. Gently simmer for 20 minutes, and then allow the mixture to cool completely before straining. Store in the refrigerator.

> ***To use:*** After washing your face, use a cotton ball to apply to affected areas.

The herbal vinegar reduces inflammation, counters infection, and fights bacteria. Also use this combination of herbs without vinegar for a cleansing facial steam. In a pinch, if you don't have an astringent on hand, apply plain witch hazel after washing your face and before moisturizing. The Burdock and Dandelion Decoction soothes inflammation and heals blemishes.

Lemongrass is an ideal astringent for toning the skin and treating acne. Brew a strong tea and apply it to the affected areas. For mild acne or the occasional outbreak, a strong infusion of chamomile can be dabbed onto the skin. A facial steam using cilantro (coriander leaves) is helpful for clearing blackheads. Additional herbs to use for acne include black cohosh, hyssop, peppermint, sage, spearmint, thyme, and yarrow. Other ingredients that help deal with acne include aloe vera, beeswax, coconut oil, and jojoba oil.

Athlete's Foot

Usually beginning between the toes, *Tinea pedis*, athlete's foot, is a fungal infection that causes an itchy, scaly rash. Other symptoms include a stinging or burning sensation. It is commonly spread in damp, moist locations such as locker rooms and showers. The infection can occur on one or both feet. Avoid scratching the rash because the infection can spread to the hands.

❁ Lemongrass and Lavender Infusion

¾ cup dried lemongrass, crumbled
¾ cup dried lavender, crumbled
2 quarts water, boiled

Place the lemongrass and lavender in a muslin bag and set aside. Bring the water to a boil in a large stockpot, and then remove it from the heat. Place the bag of herbs in the water, cover, and steep for 2 hours.

> ***To use:*** Warm the infusion to a comfortable temperature before pouring it into a foot basin. Soak the feet (or foot) for 10 to 15 minutes daily until the symptoms subside.

❁ Bay and Thyme Salve

For the infused oil:
2 teaspoons dried bay laurel, crumbled
2 teaspoons dried thyme, crumbled
½ cup coconut oil

For the salve:
½ ounce beeswax, chopped into small pieces
6–8 tablespoons infused oil

Place the bay laurel, thyme, and coconut oil in a double boiler and cover. With the heat as low as possible, warm for 20 minutes. Remove from the heat and allow it to steep for 20 minutes before straining. Place the beeswax and infused oil in a glass jar in a saucepan of water. Warm over low heat, stirring until the beeswax melts. Remove from the heat and allow it to cool completely before using or storing.

> ***To use:*** Apply to affected areas with a cotton swab several times a day or as needed.

All the herbs in the infusion and salve have analgesic, antifungal, and anti-inflammatory properties that soothe and heal athlete's foot. Coconut oil is also an antifungal and anti-inflammatory. Jojoba oil and garlic can be used to treat athlete's foot, too.

Boils and Carbuncles

Fairly common and sometimes painful, a boil is the deep-seated infection of a hair follicle or oil gland that may affect the surrounding skin. Also known as a furuncle and skin abscess, a boil most often occurs on the face, neck, armpits, thighs, and buttocks. The *Staphylococcus aureus* bacterium, commonly known as staph, is often the cause. A carbuncle is a cluster of boils that usually occurs on the neck, shoulders, and thighs.

❁ Thyme and Sage Poultice

1 tablespoon dried thyme, crumbled
1 tablespoon dried sage, crumbled
2–3 cups water

Place the thyme and sage in a muslin bag and set aside. Boil the water in a saucepan, and then remove from the heat. Place the bag of herbs in the water for 2 to 3 minutes to moisten and warm the plant material. Remove from the water and press out excess moisture.

> ***To use:*** Check that the bag of herbs is not too hot, and then set it directly on the affected area. Cover with a towel to keep it warm for as long as possible. Remove the poultice when it starts to cool.

❁ Mullein and Dandelion Compress

3 tablespoons dried mullein, crumbled
2 tablespoons dried dandelion, crumbled
2 cups water, boiled

Pre-warm a glass jar with hot tap water, and then add the mullein, dandelion, and boiled water. Cover and steep for 45 minutes before straining.

> ***To use:*** Warm to a comfortable temperature, soak a gauze pad, and then place it over the boil or carbuncle. Apply for 20 minutes, using a fresh piece of gauze every 5 minutes or so.

A poultice or compress will soothe pain and draw pus to the surface. After a boil drains, be sure to keep the area clean to avoid further infection. Beeswax used as the base for a salve or ointment will also help fight infection and heal the skin. Other herbs that can be used include burdock, lavender, and yarrow. Consult your doctor if a boil or carbuncle does not begin to heal after two or three days of herbal treatment.

Dandruff

Dandruff is a common scalp condition characterized by flaking skin. The scalp may be scaly and itchy, too. It is often aggravated during the winter when indoor heating can dry the skin. Common causes for dandruff include dry skin, oily skin that becomes irritated, not shampooing often enough, sensitivity to haircare products, and stress.

Bay Laurel Infusion

10 tablespoons dried bay laurel, crumbled
1 quart water, boiled

Pre-warm a large glass jar with hot tap water, and then add the bay laurel and boiled water. Cover and steep for 2 hours before straining.

> ***To use:*** After shampooing and rinsing, pour the infusion over your head. Massage it into the scalp. Wrap a towel around your head and leave the infusion on for 15 to 20 minutes. Rinse thoroughly.

❁ Rosemary Oil

¼ cup dried rosemary, crumbled
1 cup coconut oil

Place the rosemary and coconut oil in a double boiler and cover. With the heat as low as possible, warm for 20 minutes. Allow the oil to cool completely, and then strain.

> ***To use:*** Put a few drops on your fingertips and massage into the scalp. Wrap a towel around your head and leave the oil on for 15 minutes. Shampoo and rinse thoroughly.

A scalp massage without using oil improves blood circulation, which promotes a healthy scalp, removes dandruff, and prevents it from reforming. Additional herbs and other ingredients that can be used to control dandruff include aloe vera, burdock, chamomile, jojoba oil, olive oil, parsley, and sage. Check that the shampoo you are using is not overly drying your scalp.

Dermatitis

Dermatitis is an inflammation of the skin that causes it to become reddish, swollen, and itchy or sore. The skin may blister, ooze, or flake. There are three types of dermatitis, none of which are contagious. Contact dermatitis is caused by contact with an irritant or allergen. Seborrheic dermatitis is caused by a fungus in the skin's oil secretion. When seborrheic dermatitis occurs in infants it is called *cradle cap*. Atopic dermatitis, also known as eczema, occurs when the skin fails to protect against irritants and allergens.

❁ Lemon Balm and Nettle Ointment

For the infused oil:
1½ teaspoons dried lemon balm, crumbled
½ teaspoon dried nettle, crumbled
¼ cup coconut oil

For the ointment:
2 tablespoons cocoa butter, grated
¼ cup infused oil

Place the lemon balm, nettle, and coconut oil in a double boiler and cover. With the heat as low as possible, warm for 45 minutes. Allow it to cool slightly before straining. Combine the infused oil with the cocoa butter in a glass jar. Boil a little water in a saucepan and remove it from the heat. Place the jar in the water and stir until the cocoa butter melts. Remove the jar from the water and allow the mixture to cool to room temperature. Small particles usually appear as it cools. Boil the water again, place the jar in the water, and stir until the particles disappear. Remove the jar from the water, let the mixture cool slightly, and then place it in the refrigerator for 5 to 6 hours. After removing it from the fridge, let the mixture come to room temperature before using or storing.

> ***To use:*** Apply the ointment to affected areas several times a day.

❁ **St. John's Wort and Chamomile Bath Infusion**

2 cups dried St. John's wort, crumbled
1 cup dried chamomile, crumbled
4–5 quarts water

Bring the water to a boil in a large stockpot, and then turn off the heat. Place the St. John's wort and chamomile in a muslin bag and add it to the water. Cover and steep for 2 hours.

> ***To use:*** Warm to a comfortable temperature, and then add the infusion and herb bundle to bathwater. Soak until the water starts to cool.

The Chamomile and Lavender Gel included under Hives can also be used. When dealing with dermatitis, beeswax works well as a base ingredient in a salve or ointment.

Eczema

Eczema is the name for a group of skin conditions characterized by a red, itchy rash and dry, thickened skin. While eczema can occur at any age, it frequently appears in children. It is most commonly found on the wrists, hands, face, back of the knees, and feet. While the exact cause is unknown, eczema is thought to be caused by the immune system's overreaction to an irritant or a combination of factors that can also include environmental conditions and heredity.

❁ Nettle and Yarrow Bath Salts

For the infused oil:
1½ tablespoons dried nettle, crumbled
1½ tablespoons dried yarrow, crumbled
¾ cup coconut oil

For the bath salts:
2 cups Epsom or sea salt
2 tablespoons baking soda
¾ cup infused oil

Place the nettle, yarrow, and coconut oil in a double boiler and cover. With the heat as low as possible, warm for 45 minutes. Allow the infused oil to cool to room temperature before straining. Mix the dry ingredients together in a bowl. Slowly stir in the infused oil and mix thoroughly.

To use: Add half or all the bath salts under the running tap for a soothing soak.

❁ Lemon Balm and Peppermint Salve

For the infused oil:
3 teaspoons dried lemon balm, crumbled
1 teaspoon dried peppermint, crumbled
½ cup jojoba oil

For the salve:
7–9 tablespoons cocoa butter
6 tablespoons infused oil

Place the lemon balm, peppermint, and jojoba oil in a double boiler and cover. With the heat as low as possible, warm for 45 minutes. Remove from the heat and allow the infused oil to cool slightly before straining. Boil a little water in a saucepan and remove it from the heat. Combine the cocoa butter and infused oil in a glass jar and place it in the water. Stir until the butter melts. Remove from the water and allow the mixture to cool to room temperature. Small particles usually appear as it cools. Boil the water again, place the jar in the water, and stir until the particles disappear. Remove the jar from the water, let the mixture cool slightly, and then place it in the refrigerator for 5 to 6 hours. Allow it to come to room temperature before using or storing.

To use: Apply several times a day or as needed.

Instead of salts, a strong herbal infusion can be added to bathwater or it can be gently dabbed onto the skin. Plain witch hazel or the Burdock and Dandelion Decoction included under Acne can be used. A poultice can be used for treatment if the affected area is small. Other herbs that help soothe eczema include chamomile, lavender, rosemary, St. John's wort, and turmeric. Keep in mind that the topical use of turmeric can temporarily stain the skin. Other healing base ingredients are aloe vera and beeswax.

Hives

Medically known as urticaria, hives are characterized by swollen, pale red patches and welts on the skin that can last for minutes, hours, or days. While they are most often itchy, they can burn or sting, too. Some of the causes include food allergies, insect bites, medications, infections, and stress. Food additives can also cause a reaction.

❁ Chamomile and Lavender Gel

For the infused oil:
1 tablespoon dried chamomile, crumbled
1 tablespoon dried lavender, crumbled
½ cup coconut oil

For the gel:
6–8 tablespoons aloe vera gel
½ cup infused oil

Place the chamomile, lavender, and coconut oil in a double boiler and cover. With the heat as low as possible, warm for 30 minutes. Remove from the heat and allow the infused oil to cool completely before straining. Place the aloe vera gel in a bowl. Slowly add the oil until the gel reaches a consistency you like. Gently stir until it is thoroughly mixed. Store in a glass jar with a tight-fitting lid.

To use: Apply a light layer to affected areas several times a day or as needed.

❁ Rosemary Compress

¾ cup dried rosemary, crumbled
1 quart water, boiled

Pre-warm a large glass jar with hot tap water before adding the rosemary and boiled water. Cover and steep for 1 hour, and then strain.

To use: Soak and wring out a washcloth, and then place it over the affected area. Apply for 20 minutes, freshening the cloth every 5 minutes or so.

When the affected area is small, a cool poultice can be used. If multiple areas of the body are affected, make a strong infusion to use in a cool bath; a warm bath can exacerbate the swelling and itching. Another treatment is to apply plain witch hazel with a cotton ball. Nettle and parsley can also be used to soothe hives. At the first sign of them, a cool shower can inhibit the spread of welts.

Jock Itch

Jock itch is the common name for a fungal infection called *Tinea cruris*. It affects the skin of the genitals, inner thighs, and buttocks with an itchy or burning red rash that often forms in the shape of a ring. Other symptoms of jock itch include scaly or flaky skin and small blisters along the border of the rash.

❁ Bay and Chamomile Ointment

For the infused oil:

1 tablespoon dried bay laurel, crumbled

1 tablespoon dried chamomile, crumbled

⅓ cup coconut oil

For the ointment:
2 tablespoon cocoa butter, grated
4 tablespoons infused oil

Place the bay laurel, chamomile, and coconut oil in a double boiler and cover. With the heat as low as possible, warm for 45 minutes. Remove from the heat and allow the infused oil to cool slightly before straining. Boil a little water in a saucepan and remove it from the heat. Combine the cocoa butter and infused oil in a glass jar and place it in the water. Stir until the butter melts. Remove the jar from the water and allow the mixture to cool to room temperature. Small particles usually appear as it cools. Boil the water again, place the jar in the water, and stir until the particles disappear. Remove from the water, let it cool slightly, and then place it in the refrigerator for 5 to 6 hours. After removing from the fridge, allow the mixture to come to room temperature before using or storing.

To use: Apply a thin layer to affected areas several times a day.

❁ Lavender and Thyme Sitz Bath Infusion

1 cup dried lavender, crumbled
1 cup dried thyme, crumbled
3 quarts water

Bring the water to a boil in a large stockpot, and then turn off the heat. Place the lavender and thyme in a muslin bag and add it to the water. Cover and steep for 2 hours.

To use: Warm the infusion and add it along with the herb bag to shallow bathwater. Soak until the water begins to cool.

The herbs and coconut oil in the above recipes have antifungal and anti-inflammatory properties that soothe and heal the skin. Garlic and lemongrass can also be used for jock itch.

Psoriasis

Psoriasis is a common condition in which the life cycle of skin cells is accelerated. As they build up on the surface of the skin, they create silvery scales and red patches that can feel itchy, sore, or burning. The skin can also become dry and cracked. Most psoriasis runs in a cycle of remission and flare-up. The cause of psoriasis is unknown but is believed to be part of an immune system disorder.

❁ St. John's Wort and Dandelion Salve

For the infused oil:
½ tablespoon dried St. John's wort, crumbled
½ tablespoon dried dandelion root, chopped
½ cup jojoba oil

For the salve:
½ ounce beeswax, chopped into small pieces
6–8 tablespoons infused oil

Place the dandelion and jojoba oil in a double boiler and cover. With the heat as low as possible, warm for 40 minutes.

Remove from the heat, stir in the St. John's wort, and steep for 20 minutes before straining. Combine the beeswax and infused oil in a glass jar and place it in a saucepan of water. Warm over low heat, stirring until the beeswax melts. Remove from the heat and allow the mixture to cool completely before using or storing.

> ***To use:*** Apply a thin layer to affected areas several times a day.

❁ Angelica and Burdock Bath Salts

For the infused oil:
2 tablespoons dried angelica root, chopped
1½ tablespoons dried burdock root, chopped
¾ cup coconut oil

For the salts:
2 cups Epsom or sea salt
2 tablespoons baking soda
¾ cup infused oil

Place the angelica, burdock, and coconut oil in a double boiler and cover. With the heat as low as possible, warm for 45 minutes. Allow the infused oil to cool completely before straining. Mix the dry ingredients together in a bowl. Slowly stir in the infused oil and mix thoroughly.

> ***To use:*** Add half or all the salts under the running tap for a soothing soak.

The anti-inflammatory properties of the herbs soothe the itching and soreness while the oils and beeswax moisturize the skin. Additional herbs and other ingredients that help deal with psoriasis include aloe vera, chamomile, cocoa butter, lavender, lemon balm, turmeric, and witch hazel. The anti-inflammatory properties of witch hazel are helpful; however, when applied on its own, follow with a moisturizer.

Ringworm

Despite its name, ringworm is not caused by a worm. It is the common name for a fungal infection of the skin called *Tinea corporis*. Ringworm is characterized by an itchy, ring-shaped rash. It is highly contagious and spread by touching contaminated surfaces. When treated promptly, it clears up in three to four weeks. If it does not improve with home treatment, consult your doctor.

❁ Lemongrass and Thyme Poultice

1 tablespoon dried lemongrass, crumbled
1 tablespoon dried thyme, crumbled
2–3 cups water

Place the lemongrass and thyme in a muslin bag and set aside. Bring the water to a boil in a saucepan, and then remove it from the heat. Place the bag of herbs in the water for 2 or 3 minutes to moisten and warm the plant material. Remove from the water and press out excess moisture.

To use: Check that it's not too hot, and then set it directly on the affected area. Cover the poultice with a towel to keep it warm for as long as possible. Remove when it begins to cool. Apply 2 to 3 times a day, making a fresh poultice each time.

❁ **Garlic Oil**

1 large clove fresh garlic, crushed
1 cup coconut oil

Place the garlic clove in a small muslin bag and crush. Put the bag in a glass jar and add the coconut oil. Allow it to sit for 2 days before removing the bag of garlic.

To use: Dip a cotton swab into the oil and apply to the affected area.

With strong antifungal properties, garlic may be a bit smelly, but it is effective. Eating garlic also helps with infections. A strong tea made with burdock root or lavender can be dabbed onto the rash with a cotton swab. Turmeric can also be used for ringworm; however, it temporarily stains the skin when used topically.

Scabies

Too small to be seen by the unaided eye, the scabies mite (*Sarcoptes scabiei*) likes to nest on and under the skin. Its burrowing activities cause itching and a pimple- or blister-like rash that is often accompanied by raised lines or welts on the skin. A scabies infestation is contagious.

❁ **Anise and Bay Bath Infusion**

1½ cups aniseeds, crushed
1½ cups dried bay laurel, crumbled
4–5 quarts water

After crushing the aniseeds, combine them with the bay laurel in a muslin bag and set aside. Bring the water to a boil in a large stockpot, and then remove it from the heat. Place the bag of herbs in the water, cover, and steep for 2 hours.

To use: Warm to a comfortable temperature, and then add the infusion along with the herb bag to bathwater. Relax and soak until the water begins to cool.

❁ Lavender and Thyme Gel

For the infused oil:
1½ tablespoons dried lavender, crumbled
½ tablespoon dried thyme, crumbled
½ cup olive oil

For the gel:
6–8 tablespoons aloe vera gel
½ cup infused oil

Place the lavender, thyme, and olive oil in a double boiler and cover. With the heat as low as possible, warm for 30 minutes. Remove from the heat and allow the infused oil to cool completely before straining. Place the aloe vera gel in a bowl. Slowly add the infused oil until the gel reaches a consistency you like. Gently stir until it is thoroughly mixed. Store in a glass jar with a tight-fitting lid.

To use: Apply liberally several times a day or as needed.

Scabies can also be treated by dabbing olive oil infused with lemongrass on the affected areas. A poultice can be used on small areas. Eating garlic also helps.

Shingles

Herpes zoster, commonly known as shingles, is an infection caused by the varicella-zoster virus (VZV). It is the same virus that causes chicken pox in children that years later, if reactivated, causes shingles. While the rash can occur anywhere on the body, it most often appears first on one side of the torso. Shingles usually begins as a burning pain, numbness, or tingling sensation before producing an itchy, red rash. When blisters form, they can break open and crust over. Shingles can be spread to another person through contact with fluid from the blisters. The blisters are infectious until they dry out and crust over.

❁ Lemon Balm Tea

2 teaspoons dried lemon balm, crumbled
1 cup water, boiled

Pre-warm a cup or mug with hot tap water, and then add the lemon balm and boiled water. Cover and steep for 10 to 15 minutes before straining.

To use: Drink 2 to 3 cups a day. The tea can also be applied to the rash with a cotton ball. Cover with gauze after applying.

❁ St. John's Wort Oil

½ cup dried St. John's wort, crumbled
2 cups coconut oil

Place the St. John's wort and coconut oil in a double boiler and cover. With the heat as low as possible, warm for 30 minutes. Remove from the heat and allow the oil to cool completely before straining.

> ***To use:*** Use a cotton ball to dab a little on affected areas several times a day or as needed. Cover with gauze after applying.

In addition to topical treatment, lemon balm and St. John's wort bring relief when taken internally. Use them to make a tea or infusion and drink 2 to 3 cups a day. A small pinch of cayenne in a tablespoon of aloe vera gel can also bring relief when used topically. Test it on an area of unaffected skin to make sure it is not too strong. Do not use cayenne on areas with broken blisters. Avoid touching the rash and wash your hands frequently to prevent the spread of the virus.

Warts

Common warts are benign growths in the top layer of the skin that are caused by the human papillomavirus (HPV). The virus is contagious and can spread through contact. While they are usually skin-colored and grainy or rough, warts can also be dark and smooth. Warts are usually harmless and go away on their own.

❁ Basil Poultice

1–2 tablespoons dried basil, crumbled
jojoba oil

Place the basil in a small bowl. Warm a little bit of jojoba oil, and then add just enough to the basil to moisten it and make a thick paste.

> ***To use:*** Cover the skin with gauze and then spoon on enough of the poultice to cover the wart. Alternatively, place the poultice in a small muslin bag or tea filter bag. Use a piece of gauze to hold it in place, and then cover with a towel to keep it warm. Remove the poultice when it starts to cool. Apply 2 or 3 times a day, making a fresh poultice each time.

❁ Thyme Tincture

¾ cup dried thyme, crumbled
2 cups 80 to 100 proof alcohol (vodka, gin, brandy, or rum)

Place the thyme and alcohol in a glass jar with a tight-fitting lid. Close and shake for 1 to 2 minutes. Set aside for 2 to 3 weeks, shaking the jar every other day before straining.

> ***To use:*** Place a few drops on the wart and cover with an adhesive bandage. Apply 2 times a day.

The antiviral properties of garlic also make it useful when dealing with warts. The Garlic Oil included under Ringworm can be used or simply add the juice of 1 clove to a tablespoon of honey. Let it stand for two to three hours before applying to the wart and covering with a bandage. Adding garlic to your diet helps, too. Dabbing aloe vera gel on a wart two or three times a day is also effective.

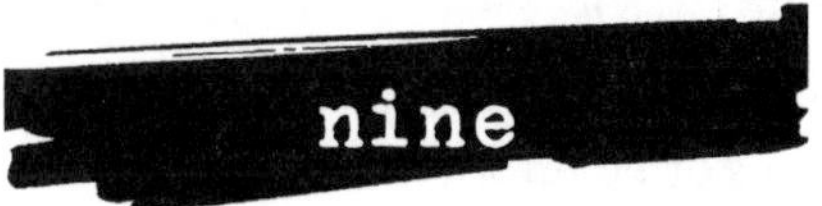

The Musculoskeletal System

The muscles and bones work together to support the body and make it possible to move. The musculoskeletal system provides shape to the body and protects vital organs. In addition to muscles and bones, this system includes tendons, cartilage, bursae, and ligaments.

Arthritis

Arthritis is the inflammation of one or more joints accompanied by pain and stiffness. The pain can come and go and ranges from mild to severe. Stiffness can sometimes decrease a joint's range of motion. Arthritis occurs when the cartilage in a joint wears away. Cartilage is a flexible connective tissue that cushions the bones. The most common type is osteoarthritis, which is also referred to as degenerative arthritis. Arthritis can also occur from traumatic stress in a joint after a fracture.

❁ Feverfew, Rosemary, and Chamomile Massage Ointment

For the infused oil:
1½ teaspoons dried feverfew, crumbled
1 teaspoon dried rosemary, crumbled
1 teaspoon dried chamomile, crumbled
½ cup coconut oil

For the ointment:
4 tablespoons cocoa butter, grated
½ cup infused oil

Place the feverfew, rosemary, chamomile, and coconut oil in a double boiler and cover. With the heat as low as possible, warm for 30 minutes. Cool slightly before straining. Combine the infused oil and cocoa butter in a glass jar. Boil a little water in a saucepan and remove it from the heat. Place the jar in the water and stir until the cocoa butter melts. Remove from the water and allow the mixture to cool to room temperature. Small particles usually appear as it cools. Boil the water again, place the jar in the water, and stir until the particles disappear. Remove from the water, let the mixture cool slightly, and then place it in the refrigerator for 5 to 6 hours. Allow it to come to room temperature before using or storing.

To use: Put a little ointment on your fingertips and gently massage affected areas.

❁ Black Cohosh and Sage Bath Infusion

1½ cups dried black cohosh, crumbled
1½ cups dried sage, crumbled
4–5 quarts water

Place the black cohosh and sage in a muslin bag and set aside. Bring the water to a boil in a large stockpot, and then remove it from the heat. Place the bag of herbs in the water, cover, and steep for 2 hours.

> ***To use:*** Warm to a comfortable temperature, and then add the infusion and the herb bag to bathwater. Soak until the water starts to cool.

Turmeric can be taken in capsule form to ease arthritis pain; the dose is usually 250 milligrams to 500 milligrams twice a day. Warm compresses also work well. Other herbs and ingredients that ease arthritis include aloe vera, angelica, bay laurel, burdock, cayenne, coriander, dandelion, dill, ginger, lemongrass, mullein, nettle, parsley, St. John's wort, thyme, and valerian. Exercising regularly and keeping the joints mobile is helpful but avoid overstressing them.

Bursitis and Tendonitis

Although these are different ailments, their treatment is the same. Occasionally, it can be difficult to tell them apart. Bursitis affects the bursae, the fluid sacs that act as cushions in the joints and aid movement. It most commonly occurs in the shoulders, knees, elbows, and hips and is caused by overuse with repetitive movement or by injury. Bursitis can sometimes be caused by infection. Symptoms can vary in their severity but typically include pain on movement, swelling, stiffness, and warmth.

Also spelled *tendinitis*, tendonitis is the irritation or inflammation of a tendon, the connective tissue that attaches muscles to bones. Tendonitis most commonly occurs in the thumbs, elbows, shoulders, knees, and heels. Although it can be caused by injury, tendonitis is usually the result of repetitive movement and occurs frequently in sports. Symptoms can include mild swelling, tenderness, pain on movement, and a dull ache just outside the joint area. An ailment known as frozen shoulder is a combination of bursitis and tendonitis.

❁ Peppermint and Rosemary Compresses

For the cool compress:
10 tablespoons dried peppermint, crumbled
1 quart water

For the warm compress:
10 tablespoons dried rosemary, crumbled
1 quart water

To make a cooling compress, place the peppermint in a prewarmed glass jar and add the boiled water. Cover, steep for 1 hour, and then strain. Place it in the refrigerator for a few minutes to chill. Follow the same steps using rosemary to make the warm compress. Strain and let it cool to a comfortable temperature; do not refrigerate.

To use: For bursitis, a cool compress should be applied the first 2 days when pain begins. After that, use a warm compress. For tendonitis, use a cool compress during the first 3 days and a warm compress after that. Soak a washcloth in the infusion, wring out, and place over the affected area. Apply for 20 minutes, freshening the cloth every 5 minutes or so.

❁ **Nettle and Mullein Liniment**

1½ tablespoons dried nettle, crumbled
1 tablespoon dried mullein, crumbled
1 cup witch hazel

Place the nettle, mullein, and witch hazel in a glass jar with a tight-fitting led. Close and shake for 1 or 2 minutes. Set aside for 4 to 6 weeks, giving the jar a good shake every day. Strain into a dark glass bottle.

To use: For bursitis, use a liniment after the first 2 days. For tendonitis, use it after the first 3 days. Place a little on your fingertips and firmly massage the affected area until the skin feels warm.

A poultice can be used in place of a warm compress. Use a muslin bag to hold the plant material and place it over the affected area. Cover the poultice with a towel to keep it warm. Turmeric can be taken in capsule form to ease the pain; the dose is usually 250 milligrams to 500 milligrams twice a day. Other herbs and ingredients that can ease bursitis and tendonitis include aloe vera, cayenne, ginger, and lemongrass. Rest is also helpful in healing these conditions.

Carpal Tunnel Syndrome

Carpal tunnel syndrome is a condition characterized by tingling, numbness, and pain in the fingers and hand. The sensation sometimes travels from the wrist up the arm. It is caused when a nerve is compressed in the narrow passageway called the *carpal tunnel*, located on the palm side of the wrist. This condition can also cause weakness in the hand.

❁ Cayenne Rubbing Oil

1 teaspoon cayenne, powdered
½ cup olive oil

Start with ½ teaspoon of cayenne and mix well with the olive oil. Test on a small area of skin. If you don't feel any warming effects, increase the amount of cayenne and test again. It is important to mix and test slowly to get the ratio that works best for you and to avoid burning the skin.

To use: Put a little of the oil on your fingertips and gently massage the affected area.

❁ Bay and Chamomile Compress

6 tablespoons dried bay laurel, crumbled
4 tablespoons dried chamomile, crumbled
1 quart water, boiled

Pre-warm a large glass jar with hot tap water before adding the bay, chamomile, and boiled water. Cover and steep for 1 hour, and then strain.

To use: Warm to a comfortable temperature. Soak and wring out a washcloth, and then place it over the afflicted area. Apply for 20 minutes, freshening the cloth every 5 minutes or so.

Sage and St. John's wort can also be used topically. Turmeric can be taken in capsule form to ease carpal tunnel pain; the dose is usually 250 milligrams to 500 milligrams twice a day. When working at a computer, it is important to maintain good posture and take frequent breaks to exercise and stretch your fingers, hands, and wrists. Experiment with different computer keyboards and wrist rests to find a setup that works best for you.

Gout

Also known as gouty arthritis, gout is the painful inflammation that occurs when uric acid forms needle-like crystal deposits in the joints. Uric acid is created during the breakdown of some foods, but it is usually dissolved in the blood and released from the body in urine. Crystal deposits are formed when there is a high level of uric acid in the blood. Gout most often appears in the knee, ankle, foot, and big toe. Attacks of gout can occur suddenly and often at night. Symptoms include swelling, stiffness, severe pain, and redness. Drinking alcohol can trigger gout attacks.

❁ Nettle Tea

2 teaspoons dried nettle leaves, crumbled
1 cup water, boiled

Pre-warm a cup or mug with hot tap water, and then add the nettle and boiled water. Cover and steep for 10 to 15 minutes before straining.

To use: Drink up to 3 cups a day during gout attacks.

❁ Mullein and Burdock Compress

6 tablespoons dried mullein root, chopped
4 tablespoons dried burdock root, chopped
1 quart water

Place the mullein, burdock, and water in a saucepan and bring to a boil. Reduce the heat to as low as possible, cover, and gently simmer for 20 minutes. Remove from the heat and steep for 15 minutes before straining.

To use: Soak and wring out a washcloth, and then place it over the affected joint. Apply for 20 minutes, freshening the cloth every 5 minutes or so. The compress can be applied warm or cool.

Bath salts made with Epsom salt and an herbal infusion or Epsom salt on its own helps reduce inflammation and pain. Turmeric can be taken in capsule form to ease the pain; the dose is usually 250 milligrams to 500 milligrams twice a day. Other herbs that help ease gout include angelica, cayenne, dandelion, ginger, and parsley. Drinking eight or more glasses of water a day helps flush uric acid from the body.

Low Back Pain

Known as lumbago in the past, low back pain occurs in the lumbar region of the spine. Located between the rib cage and sacrum (bottom of the spine), these five vertebrae are especially important for structural support and movement. Low back pain can be sharp or dull, intermittent or constant, and it may extend from the back to the buttocks or hips. It often gets better on its own. Low back pain can be caused by overactivity, heavy lifting, vigorous exercise or sports, sitting for long periods with inadequate back support, poor posture, and a herniated disc. If low back pain occurs after a fall or injury, see your doctor right away, especially if there is numbness or weakness in the legs.

❁ Ginger Compress

¾ cup fresh ginger, chopped
1 quart water

Place the ginger and water in a saucepan and bring to a boil. Reduce the heat, cover, and gently simmer for 30 minutes. Allow it to cool to a comfortable temperature, and then strain.

> ***To use:*** Soak and wring out a washcloth, and then place it over the lower back. Cover the compress with a towel to keep it warm and hold it in place. Freshen the cloth by dipping it in the infusion every 5 minutes or so.

❁ Feverfew and Black Cohosh Tincture

½ cup dried feverfew, crumbled
¼ cup dried black cohosh, crumbled
2 cups 80 to 100 proof alcohol (vodka, gin, brandy, or rum)

Place the feverfew, black cohosh, and alcohol in a glass jar with a tight-fitting lid. Close and shake for 1 to 2 minutes. Set aside for 2 to 3 weeks, shaking the jar every other day. Strain and store in a dark glass bottle.

To use: Add 1 teaspoon to a cup of juice, tea, or water. Alternatively, take ½ to 1 teaspoon straight 2 times a day.

Other treatments include a warm bath with an herbal infusion, an infused oil for massage, and fomentation, the alternating of warm and cool compresses. Turmeric can be taken in capsule form to ease low back pain; the dose is usually 250 milligrams to 500 milligrams twice a day. The Cayenne Rubbing Oil included under Carpal Tunnel Syndrome also works well. At bedtime, valerian tea aids general muscle relaxation. Other herbs to use for low back pain include mullein, rosemary, spearmint, and thyme. Gentle exercise and stretching are helpful, too.

Muscle Soreness or Stiffness

Common muscle soreness and stiffness is usually localized to one or a few muscles. Sore, tight muscles can often make it difficult to move. Some of the causes include overuse, minor injury, muscle tension, and stress. Muscle stiffness can also occur after inactivity.

❁ Bay and Lavender Bath Salts

For the infused oil:

2 tablespoons dried bay laurel, crumbled

2 tablespoons dried lavender, crumbled

2 cups coconut oil

For the salts:
4 cups Epsom salt
4 tablespoons baking soda (optional)
¾ cup infused oil

Place the bay, lavender, and coconut oil in a double boiler and cover. With the heat as low as possible, warm for 20 minutes. Remove from the heat and allow the infused oil to cool completely before straining. Combine the dry ingredients in a bowl. Slowly stir in the infused oil and mix thoroughly.

To use: Add half or all the bath salts under the running tap for a soothing soak.

❁ Coriander and Ginger Massage Oil

3 tablespoons coriander seeds, crushed
2 tablespoons fresh ginger, coarsely grated
2 cups coconut oil

After crushing the coriander seeds, combine them with the ginger and coconut oil in a double boiler and cover. With the heat as low as possible, warm for 40 minutes. Allow the oil to cool completely before straining.

To use: Place a little oil on your fingertips and firmly massage sore muscles.

The anti-inflammatory properties of the herbs and the minerals in Epsom salt help relax muscles and relieve soreness. A warm compress made with an herbal infusion is especially helpful for muscles that are sore after a workout. A cool compress may not relieve pain, but it reduces stiffness and restores range of motion. Chamomile or valerian tea at bedtime helps, too. Other herbs to use for sore or stiff muscles include cayenne, feverfew, hyssop, lemongrass, mullein, nettle, oregano, peppermint, rosemary, sage, spearmint, St. John's wort, thyme, and yarrow.

Muscle Spasm and Cramp

A spasm is the sudden involuntary contraction of one or more muscles that does not last long. A muscle cramp is a sustained spasm. When a spasm or cramp occurs in the leg, it is often referred to as a charley horse. The pain can range from mild to severe but usually resolves on its own. Some of the causes for muscle spasm and cramp include a reaction to pain, overexertion, fatigue, and dehydration. See your doctor if they last a long time, are extremely severe, or frequently recur.

❁ Black Cohosh Tea

1–2 teaspoons dried black cohosh, crumbled
1 cup water, boiled

Pre-warm a cup or mug with hot tap water, and then add the black cohosh and boiled water. Cover and steep for 10 minutes before straining.

To use: Sweeten to taste and drink 1 cup following an episode of muscle spasm or cramp.

❁ **Rosemary and Thyme Compress**

5 tablespoons dried rosemary, crumbled
5 tablespoons dried thyme, crumbled
1 quart water, boiled

Pre-warm a large glass jar, and then add the rosemary, thyme, and boiled water. Cover and steep for 1 hour before straining.

> ***To use:*** Warm to a comfortable temperature, soak and wring out a washcloth, and then place it over the affected area. Apply for 15 to 20 minutes, freshening the cloth every 5 minutes or so.

Other herbs to use include cayenne, chamomile, coriander, peppermint, and valerian. Massage and gentle stretching also help relieve a muscle spasm or cramp.

Rheumatoid Arthritis

Rheumatoid arthritis is a type of inflammatory arthritis where the immune system mistakenly attacks the joints. The exact cause is unknown, but current thought is that it may happen because of a combination of genetic and environmental triggers. Symptoms of rheumatoid arthritis include pain, stiffness, swelling, and limited motion in the joints.

❁ **Aloe and Ginger Gel**

For the infused oil:
2 tablespoons fresh ginger, coarsely grated
⅓ cup olive oil

For the gel:
3–4 tablespoons aloe vera gel
¼ cup infused oil

Place the ginger in a small muslin bag in a double boiler with the olive oil and cover. With the heat as low as possible, warm for 45 minutes. Remove from the heat and allow the infused oil to cool completely. Squeeze excess oil out of the muslin bag. Place the aloe gel in a bowl. Slowly add the oil until it reaches a consistency you like. Stir until it is thoroughly mixed. Store in a glass jar with a tight-fitting lid.

To use: Place a little on your fingertips and gently massage sore joints.

❁ Yarrow and Nettle Salve

For the infused oil:
2 teaspoons dried yarrow, crumbled
1½ teaspoons dried nettle, crumbled
½ cup olive oil

For the salve:
3 tablespoons cocoa butter, grated
½ cup infused oil

Place the yarrow, nettle, and olive oil in a double boiler and cover. With the heat as low as possible, warm for 20 minutes. Remove from the heat and steep for 20 minutes before straining. Combine the infused oil and cocoa butter in a glass jar. Boil a little water in a saucepan and remove it from the heat. Place the jar in the water and stir until the cocoa butter melts. Remove from the water and allow it to cool to room temperature. Small particles usually appear as it cools. Boil the water again, place the jar in the water, and stir until the particles disappear. Remove from the water, let the mixture cool slightly, and then place it in the refrigerator for 5 to 6 hours. Allow it to come to room temperature before using or storing.

To use: Place a little on your fingertips and gently massage affected joints.

The Cayenne Rubbing Oil included under Carpal Tunnel Syndrome can be used for rheumatoid arthritis, too. Adding ginger and turmeric to the diet can help reduce inflammation. Warm compresses and baths also help. Other herbs to use for rheumatoid arthritis include black cohosh, chamomile, dandelion, feverfew, and valerian.

Sciatica

Sciatica is pain or numbness that runs from the lower back down the leg along the pathway of the sciatic nerve, which is the longest nerve in the body. It typically affects only one side of the body and occurs when the sciatic nerve is compressed. Some of the causes include a herniated disc, injury, muscle strain, arthritis in the spine, sacroiliac joint dysfunction, and degenerative disc disease.

❁ St. John's Wort Liniment

2½ tablespoons dried St. John's wort, crumbled
1 cup witch hazel

Place the St. John's wort and witch hazel in a glass jar with a tight-fitting lid. Close and shake for 1 or 2 minutes. Set aside for 4 to 6 weeks, giving the jar a good shake every day. Strain into a dark glass bottle.

> ***To use:*** Place a little on your fingertips and firmly massage the affected area until the skin feels warm.

❁ Lemon Balm and Bay Bath Infusion

2 cups dried lemon balm, crumbled
1 cup dried bay laurel, crumbled
4–5 quarts water

Place the lemon balm and bay laurel in a muslin bag and set aside. Bring the water to a boil in a large stockpot, and then remove it from the heat. Place the bag of herbs in the water, cover, and steep for 2 hours.

> ***To use:*** Warm the infusion to a comfortable temperature. Add the infusion and the bag of herbs to bathwater for a soothing soak.

Warm compresses and massaging with herb-infused oil also help relieve sciatica. Valerian tea or capsules at bedtime aids general muscle relaxation. Other herbs to use for sciatica include burdock, cayenne, chamomile, ginger, lavender, and thyme.

Shin Splints

Medically known as medial tibial stress syndrome, shin splints occur as pain along the shin bone (tibia) at the front of the leg below the knee. Although it most often happens to athletes, it can happen to runners or anyone who may overwork the muscles and put excessive strain on the tendons of the lower leg. Shin splints can also be caused by wearing inappropriate or worn-out footwear, running on a slanted surface, or frequent starting and stopping movement as when playing basketball.

❁ Thyme and Chamomile Tincture

3 tablespoons dried thyme, crumbled
3 tablespoons dried chamomile, crumbled
1 cup 80 to 100 proof alcohol (vodka, gin, brandy, or rum)

Place the thyme, chamomile, and alcohol in a glass jar with a tight-fitting lid. Close and shake for 1 to 2 minutes, and then set aside. Shake the jar every other day for 2 to 4 weeks, and then strain. Store in a dark glass bottle.

To use: Add 1 teaspoon to a cup of tea, water, or fruit juice. Take 2 or 3 times a day.

❁ Dandelion and Lemongrass Massage Oil

3 tablespoons dried dandelion root, coarsely chopped
2 tablespoons dried lemongrass, crumbled
2 cups coconut oil

Place the dandelion and coconut oil in a double boiler and cover. With the heat as low as possible, warm for 30 minutes. Remove from the heat, add the lemongrass, and steep for 20 minutes before straining.

To use: Use massage after the first 48 hours. Place a little oil on your fingertips and gently massage the affected area.

The antispasmodic properties of thyme and chamomile are especially good to soothe the pain of shin splints. They can be taken as an infusion or strong tea. For topical treatments, use a cold compress for the first forty-eight hours, and then alternate warm and cold treatments. The Cayenne Rubbing Oil included under Carpal Tunnel Syndrome works well as a warm treatment. Other herbs to use for shin splints include anise, black cohosh, feverfew, and ginger.

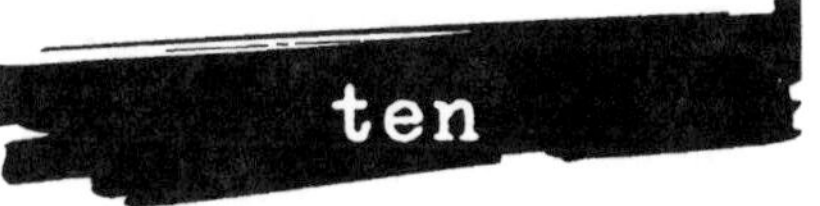

The Nervous System

The nervous system can be thought of as the body's electrical wiring and communications system. In addition to sensory neurons, it has specialized cells that transmit signals between various parts of the body. Controlling everything from the heartbeat to emotions, the system has two divisions: The central nervous system consists of the brain and spinal cord. The peripheral nervous system consists of all the nerves outside of the brain and spine. The function of the peripheral nervous system is to connect everything in the body with the central nervous system.

Insomnia and Sleep

Insomnia is defined as having difficulty falling asleep, staying asleep, or waking up early and being unable to get back to sleep. It can be caused by stress, life events, a changing work schedule, jet lag, and eating too much before bed. It is not unusual for insomnia to happen from time to time. Even though it often sorts itself out, the symptoms of low energy, fatigue, moodiness, and trouble concentrating can be difficult to deal with.

Chronic insomnia is defined as occurring at least three times a week for more than three weeks. It can last for months or years. Some of the causes for chronic insomnia include medications, a medical condition, caffeine, nicotine, and alcohol.

❁ Valerian and Lavender Tincture

1 cup dried valerian, chopped
¼ cup dried lavender, crumbled
2 cups 80 to 100 proof alcohol (vodka, gin, brandy, or rum)

Place the valerian, lavender, and alcohol in a glass jar with a tight-fitting lid. Close and shake for 1 to 2 minutes. Shake every other day for 2 to 4 weeks, and then strain. Store in a dark glass bottle.

> ***To use:*** Pre-warm a cup or mug with hot tap water, and then add 1 teaspoon of tincture and 1 cup of boiling water. Wait about 5 minutes for the alcohol in the tincture to evaporate. Drink an hour before going to bed. Take a smaller dose of ½ teaspoon the first time you try valerian.

❁ Anise and Milk

1 teaspoon aniseeds, crushed
1 cup milk

Lightly toast the aniseeds in a dry frying pan before crushing, and then place them in a pre-warmed cup. Heat the milk to just below the boiling point and pour it over the seeds. Allow it to cool to a drinkable temperature before straining.

To use: Add a little honey to taste. Drink about half an hour before going to bed.

Valerian is an excellent sleep aid and those who brave its bitter taste swear by it. Another effective method for taking valerian is by capsule. A standard dose is between 400 milligrams to 900 milligrams; however, try the smaller dose first. Valerian works well with lemon balm when dealing with insomnia.

Lavender is most widely known for its calming and soothing properties. A little sleep pillow or muslin bag stuffed with lavender can add a relaxing touch for bedtime. Put the pillow in the microwave just long enough to warm the lavender and release more of its scent. St. John's wort tea improves the quality of sleep and is especially soothing with chamomile. Other herbs that aid restful sleep include angelica, basil, coriander, dill, mullein, oregano, peppermint, sage, and spearmint.

Mental Fatigue

Mental fatigue is a sign that our brains are saying, "Whoa, slow down." It usually results when we feel overwhelmed with too much to do, too many decisions to make, and too many demands on us. Some of the symptoms include irritability, impatience, physical fatigue without cause, and a lack of concentration.

❁ Rosemary and Lemongrass Tea

1 teaspoon dried rosemary, crumbled
1 teaspoon dried lemongrass, crumbled
1 cup water, boiled

Pre-warm a cup or mug with hot tap water, and then add the rosemary, lemongrass, and boiled water. Cover and steep for 10 to 15 minutes before straining.

To use: Drink 2 to 4 cups a day.

❁ Ginger and Nettle Decoction

2 tablespoons dried ginger, chopped
2 tablespoons dried nettle root, chopped
1 quart water

Place the ginger, nettle, and water in a saucepan and bring to a boil. Stir, cover, and reduce the heat to as low as possible. Simmer for 25 minutes, and then allow it to cool completely before straining. Store in the refrigerator.

To use: Warm and drink a cup at a time. Take 2 to 3 cups a day.

Lemongrass, ginger, and nettle promote mental clarity and focus. Widely known as a tonic for the nerves, rosemary can help lift mental fog. Use ½ teaspoon of rosemary tincture in a cup of water or juice. A strong cup of peppermint tea is also helpful. Other herbs to use for mental fatigue include basil, coriander, feverfew, sage, and valerian. To aid recovery, be sure to take lunches and short breaks. Take a few minutes to simply look out the window and have a cup of tea. Also, get physical exercise every day.

Motion Sickness

Symptoms of motion sickness can include a queasy stomach, dizziness, vomiting, and cold sweat. It can occur with any type of transportation and is the same as seasickness and travel sickness. The current theory points to the vestibular system, which is a part of the nervous system located in the inner ear. The vestibular system deals with balance, movement, and spatial orientation. With motion sickness, conflicting sensory signals are sent to the brain saying that you are sitting still and that you are moving at the same time. The cause for this is unknown.

❁ Mint Tea

2–4 teaspoons dried peppermint or spearmint, crumbled
2 cups water, boiled

Pre-warm a cup or mug with hot tap water, and then add the mint and boiled water. Cover and steep for 10 to 15 minutes before straining.

> ***To use:*** Take the tea along with you in a thermos and drink ½ cup at a time or slowly sip during travel.

❁ Ginger and Turmeric Syrup

2 tablespoons dried ginger, chopped
2 tablespoons dried turmeric, chopped
2 cups water
½ cup honey

Combine the ginger, turmeric, and water in a saucepan, cover, and bring to a boil. Reduce the heat to as low as possible and simmer at least 30 minutes or until the volume is reduced by half. Strain out the herbs, return 1 cup of liquid to the saucepan, and add the honey. Warm on low heat, stirring until the mixture is smooth. Remove from the heat, allow the mixture to cool slightly, and then pour into a glass jar with a tight-fitting lid. Store in the refrigerator where it will keep for several weeks.

To use: Take 1 teaspoon as needed.

Other herbs that ease motion sickness include basil, cayenne, chamomile, fennel, and oregano. During travel, it helps avoid reading or using electronic devices and to focus your gaze on a stationary object. Stay hydrated before and during travel and avoid heavy, greasy foods.

Nerve Pain

While neuropathic or nerve pain seems to occur for no obvious reason, it is usually caused by damaged nerves sending scrambled messages to the brain. Nerve damage can result from a physical injury, chemotherapy, or a disease such as diabetes, Lyme disease, and hepatitis B or C. Symptoms vary but can include numbness, tingling, burning, and electric sensations. It is important to consult your doctor and coordinate your at-home care.

❁ St. John's Wort and Lemon Balm Massage Ointment

For the infused oil:
2 teaspoons dried St. John's wort, crumbled
1½ teaspoons dried lemon balm, crumbled
½ cup coconut oil

For the ointment:
4 tablespoons cocoa butter, grated
½ cup infused oil

Place the St. John's wort, lemon balm, and coconut oil in a double boiler and cover. With the heat as low as possible, warm for 30 minutes. Allow it to cool slightly before straining. Combine the cocoa butter and infused oil in a glass jar. Boil a little water in a saucepan and remove it from the heat. Place the jar in the water and stir until the cocoa butter melts. Remove it from the water and allow the mixture to cool to room temperature. Small particles usually appear as it cools. Boil the water again, place the jar in the water, and stir until the particles disappear. Remove from the water, let the mixture cool slightly, and then place it in the refrigerator for 5 to 6 hours. Allow the mixture to come to room temperature before using or storing.

To use: Put a little on your fingertips and gently massage the affected areas.

❁ Angelica and Coriander Infusion

3 tablespoons angelica seeds, crushed
2 tablespoons coriander seeds, crushed
1 quart water, boiled

Lightly toast the angelica and coriander seeds in a dry frying pan before crushing. Pre-warm a large glass jar with hot tap water, and then add the seeds and boiled water. Cover and steep for 45 to 50 minutes, and then strain. Store in the refrigerator.

To use: Warm a cup at a time and drink 2 to 3 cups a day.

Lemon balm and St. John's wort strengthen the nervous system and, in addition to topical use, they can be taken as a tea or an infusion. The Cayenne Rubbing Oil included under Carpal Tunnel Syndrome in Chapter 9 is also effective for easing nerve pain. Other herbs to use include chamomile, ginger, peppermint, turmeric, and valerian.

Nervous Tension

Nervous tension is the body's reaction to emotional upsets, stress, and anxiety. While symptoms may vary, they can include muscle tension, rapid heartbeat, upset stomach, nausea, sweaty hands, hot or cold flushes, and restlessness.

❁ Peppermint, Mullein, and Feverfew Tea

1 teaspoon dried peppermint, crumbled
½ teaspoon dried mullein, crumbled
½ teaspoon dried feverfew, crumbled
1 cup water, boiled

Pre-warm a cup or mug with hot tap water, and then add the peppermint, mullein, feverfew, and boiled water. Cover and steep for 10 to 15 minutes before straining.

To use: Drink 2 to 3 cups a day.

❁ Lavender and Sage Bath Infusion

2 cups dried lavender, crumbled
1 cup dried sage, crumbled
4–5 quarts water

Place the lavender and sage in a muslin bag and set aside. Bring the water to a boil in a large stockpot, and then remove it from the heat. Place the bag of herbs in the water, cover, and steep for 2 hours.

To use: Warm the infusion to a comfortable temperature before adding it and the bag of herbs to your bathwater for a soothing soak in the tub.

A tincture of hyssop is another way to deal with nervous tension. Take ½ to 1 teaspoon 2 to 3 times a day. Hyssop also serves as a tonic to support the nervous system. Use lavender to make an infused oil to massage tense muscles or the temples, which aids relaxation. Other herbs to use for nervous tension include angelica, basil, chamomile, coriander, dill, lemon balm, lemongrass, oregano, rosemary, St. John's wort, and valerian.

In addition to physical exercise such as a brisk walk, take breaks and focus on deep, slow breathing. Also take time to relax. Make the process of preparing tea a time to unwind.

Postpartum Blues

During one of the happiest times in our lives, the "baby blues" can be a surprise. It can include symptoms such as anxiety, mood swings, crying, sadness, and trouble sleeping. Don't feel embarrassed because it happens to many of us and it's no wonder with all the physical and hormonal changes that take place in the body during and after pregnancy. If the symptoms are severe or last more than a couple weeks, speak with your doctor because you may have postpartum depression, which is more serious and should be treated professionally.

❁ Chamomile and Anise Infusion

3 tablespoons dried chamomile, crumbled
2 tablespoons aniseeds, crushed
1 quart water, boiled

Lightly toast the aniseeds in a dry frying pan over low heat before crushing. Pre-warm a large glass jar with hot tap water, and then add the seeds, chamomile, and boiled water. Cover and steep for 30 minutes before straining. Store in the refrigerator.

To use: Warm a cup at a time. Drink up to 3 cups a day.

❁ Dill and Caraway Tea

1 teaspoon dillseeds, crushed
1 teaspoon caraway seeds, crushed
1 cup water, boiled

Lightly toast the dill and caraway seeds in a dry frying pan over low heat before crushing. Pre-warm a cup or mug with hot tap water, and then add the seeds and boiled water. Cover and steep for 10 to 15 minutes before straining.

To use: Drink 1 to 2 cups a day.

In addition to helping with postpartum blues, dill, anise, caraway, and fennel also support lactation by building a sufficient milk supply. If you are not nursing, lemon balm and St. John's wort can help you through the blues.

Seasonal Affective Disorder (SAD)

Seasonal affective disorder is a type of depression that usually occurs in the winter; however, it can appear during the summer for some people. Symptoms include moodiness, low energy, problems sleeping, a change in appetite, and difficulty concentrating. The cause is unknown.

❁ St. John's Wort and Lemon Balm Tincture

6 tablespoons dried St. John's wort, crumbled
6 tablespoons dried lemon balm, crumbled
2 cups 80 to 100 proof alcohol (vodka, gin, brandy, or rum)

Place the St. John's wort, lemon balm, and alcohol in a glass jar with a tight-fitting lid. Close and shake for 1 to 2 minutes, and then set aside. Shake the jar every other day for 2 to 4 weeks, and then strain. Store in a dark glass bottle.

To use: Take ½ to 1 teaspoon 2 times a day for a 3-week period. Stop taking it for 1 week, and then repeat if necessary.

❁ Lemon Balm Tea

2 teaspoons dried lemon balm, crumbled
1 cup water, boiled

Pre-warm a cup or mug with hot tap water, and then add the lemon balm and boiled water. Cover and steep for 10 to 15 minutes before straining.

To use: Drink 2 to 3 cups a day.

Restorative for the nervous system, St. John's wort is not an instant cure and usually takes a couple weeks for its effect to become apparent. Lemon balm is calming and supports a healthy nervous system.

Stress and Anxiety

Stress and anxiety share many symptoms, such as muscle tension, rapid heartbeat, and headache. It can be difficult to tell them apart as both can result in a lack of focus, sleeplessness, excessive worry, irritability, and exhaustion.

Stress is a normal reaction and part of the nervous system's fight-or-flight response, telling the body that it has to step up to the plate and do something. Sometimes the body stays on high alert, making us feel overwhelmed, which can lead to other problems.

Occasional anxiety is also normal. It can be a reaction to stress, or it can arise when the source of stress is not clear. Its hallmarks are excessive worry and stress that is out of proportion to an anticipated event or the potential outcome of an event or situation.

❁ Basil, Lemon Balm, and Chamomile Infusion

2 tablespoons dried basil, crumbled
2 tablespoons dried lemon balm, crumbled
1 tablespoon dried chamomile, crumbled
1 quart water, boiled

Pre-warm a large jar with hot tap water, and then add the basil, lemon balm, chamomile, and boiled water. Cover and steep for 35 minutes before straining. Store in the refrigerator.

To use: Warm and drink a cup at a time. Take up to 3 or 4 cups a day.

❁ Lavender and Rosemary Bath Salts

For the infused oil:
1½ tablespoons dried lavender, crumbled
1½ tablespoons dried rosemary, crumbled
¾ cup coconut oil

For the salts:
2 cups Epsom or sea salt
2 tablespoons baking soda (optional)
¾ cup infused oil

Place the lavender, rosemary, and coconut oil in a double boiler and cover. With the heat as low as possible, warm for

40 minutes. Allow the infused oil to cool completely. Combine the dry ingredients in a bowl. Slowly stir in the infused oil and mix thoroughly.

> ***To use:*** Add half or all the bath salts under the running tap for a soothing soak.

Chamomile, lavender, lemon balm, and rosemary are known for combatting stress. Basil has mild sedative properties and is considered a tonic that supports the nervous system. Instead of an infusion, try a tincture. Use 1 teaspoon in a cup of water, tea, or fruit juice two to three times a day. Lemon balm works well with valerian when dealing with stress.

When taking a soothing bath, add a handful of rose petals to the water for an extra aromatic treat. Other herbs to use for stress and anxiety include angelica, anise, coriander, ginger, hyssop, lemongrass, spearmint, and St. John's wort.

When feeling stressed, relaxation and breathing exercises or doing something creative can help. Physical activity and exercise are helpful for both stress and anxiety. Keeping a healthy diet, avoiding alcohol and caffeine, and seeking professional help are especially important if anxiety persists.

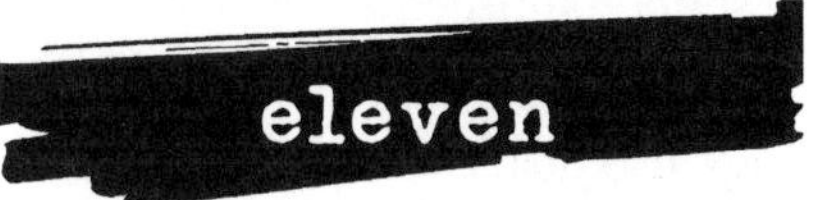

The Reproductive System

While the primary function of this system is to make babies, the hormones produced in the ovaries and testes influence bones, skin, elimination, moods, and more. While the majority of issues that can be treated with home remedies are centered on menstruation and menopause, there are a few others that herbs can help.

Breastfeeding

Breastfeeding has many benefits for your baby. All the nutrients a baby requires during the first six months are contained in breast milk. It aids in the baby's brain development and helps build their immune system. Breastfeeding also establishes an important bond between mother and child. Although it is the most natural way to feed your baby, it is not without a few challenges.

Increase Breast Milk

Produced on a supply-and-demand basis, the best way to increase breast milk is to nurse your baby more often. Pumping between feedings also helps.

❁ Caraway and Dill Infusion

3 tablespoons caraway seeds, crushed
3 tablespoons dillseeds, crushed
1 quart water, boiled

Lightly toast the caraway and dillseeds in a dry frying pan over low heat before crushing. Pre-warm a large glass jar with hot tap water, and then add the seeds and boiled water. Cover and steep for 30 minutes before straining. Store in the refrigerator.

> ***To use:*** Warm and drink a cup at a time. Take up to 3 cups a day.

Caraway and dill are warming herbs that increase the flow of breast milk. They help ease postpartum baby blues, too. Both seeds and leaves of the dill plant help increase lactation; however, the seeds are more potent. In addition to increasing milk supply, dill functions as a treatment for breast congestion that sometimes occurs during nursing. Dill tea taken by nursing mothers also helps relieve colic in their babies. Other herbs that help increase the flow of breast milk are anise and fennel.

Postweaning

Just as nursing more often increases breast milk, gradually reducing feeding at the breast decreases the supply.

❁ Sage Tea

½ teaspoon dried sage, crumbled
1 cup water, boiled

Pre-warm a cup or mug with hot tap water, and then add the sage and boiled water. Cover and steep for 10 to 15 minutes before straining.

To use: Drink up to 3 cups a day.

The drying properties of sage make it effective for reducing the production of breast milk. Parsley can also be used to help dry up milk after weaning.

Mastitis

Mastitis is the inflammation of breast tissue that sometimes includes infection. It often occurs in women who are breastfeeding due to a blocked milk duct. It can also be caused by bacteria. The inflammation is usually accompanied by pain, swelling, warmth, and redness. Other symptoms may include fever and chills. Mastitis can also occur in women who are not nursing and in men.

❁ Chamomile Poultice

4 tablespoons dried chamomile, crumbled
2–3 cups water

Place the chamomile in a muslin bag and set aside. Bring the water to a boil in a saucepan, and then remove it from the heat. Place the bag of herbs in the water for 2 to 3 minutes to moisten and warm the plant material. Remove from the water and press out excess moisture.

> ***To use:*** Check that it is not too hot, and then set the poultice on the affected area. Cover with a towel to keep it warm for as long as possible. Remove when it starts to cool. Apply several times a day, making a fresh poultice each time.

❁ Dandelion and Ginger Compress

3 tablespoons dried dandelion root, finely chopped
2 tablespoons dried ginger, finely chopped
1 quart water, boiled

Pre-warm a large glass jar, and then add the dandelion, ginger, and boiled water. Cover and steep for 2 hours before straining.

> ***To use:*** Warm to a comfortable temperature. Soak and wring out a washcloth, and then place it over the affected area. Apply for 20 minutes, freshening the cloth every 5 minutes or so.

As an alternative to the poultice, a chamomile tea bag can be used; warm it in a cup of hot water for a few minutes before applying. A poultice or compress is effective for sore nipples, too. Aloe vera, parsley, and St. John's wort can also be used to ease mastitis.

Menopause

Menopause is a natural process that marks the end of menstruation. It occurs in three stages: perimenopause, menopause, and postmenopause. Also referred to as menopause transition, perimenopause can occur years before menopause. Postmenopause can extend for years afterward. The time frame for these stages and the symptoms can vary widely. Symptoms may include hot flashes and night sweats, chills, digestive problems, fatigue, headaches, muscle aches, sleep problems, and mood swings.

General Discomforts

Whether or not you have the classic symptoms or just feel out of sorts, taking time to care for yourself can make a huge difference in your overall health and well-being.

❁ Fennel and St. John's Wort Tea

1½ teaspoons fennel seeds, crushed
½ teaspoon dried St. John's wort, crumbled
1 cup water, boiled

Lightly toast the fennel seeds in a dry frying pan over low heat before crushing. Pre-warm a cup or mug with hot tap water, and then add the fennel seeds, St. John's wort, and boiled water. Cover and steep for 10 to 15 minutes before straining.

> ***To use:*** Drink 2 to 3 cups a day. Use St. John's wort on a daily basis for a 3-week period, and then stop for 1 week before using it again.

❁ Lemon Balm and Thyme Infusion

3 tablespoons dried lemon balm, crumbled
2 tablespoons dried thyme, crumbled
1 quart water, boiled

Pre-warm a large glass jar with hot tap water, and then add the lemon balm, thyme, and boiled water. Cover and steep for 35 minutes before straining. Store in the refrigerator.

> ***To use:*** Warm and drink a cup at a time. Take 3 to 4 cups a day.

Fennel has a toning effect on women's reproductive systems and is helpful before, during, and after menopause. In addition to general discomforts, black cohosh is helpful for hormone-related headaches and migraines and, when combined with aloe vera, is effective for relieving vaginal dryness. Other herbs that relieve discomforts include anise, chamomile, lavender, nettle, sage, and valerian.

Hot Flashes and Night Sweats

The change in estrogen levels before, during, and after menopause affects the body's thermostat, producing sudden intense heat during any time of day and heavy sweating at night.

❁ Black Cohosh Decoction

4 tablespoons black cohosh, chopped
1 quart water

Place the black cohosh and water in a saucepan and bring to a boil. Stir, cover, and reduce the heat to as low as possible. Simmer for 30 minutes, and then allow the mixture to cool completely before straining. Store in the refrigerator.

> ***To use:*** Warm and drink a cup at a time. Because black cohosh has a bitter taste, you may want to sweeten it with honey or sugar. Take 1 to 2 times a day.

❁ Spearmint Spray

7 teaspoons dried spearmint, crumbled
2 cups water, boiled

Pre-warm a glass jar with hot tap water, and then add the spearmint and boiled water. Cover and steep for 20 to 25 minutes. Allow it to cool to room temperature before straining.

> ***To use:*** Pour the infusion into a spray bottle with a fine-mist nozzle. Spritz your face, arms, and legs as needed.

Spearmint is used for the spray because it is especially cooling to the skin. To avoid its taste, black cohosh can be taken in capsules. Other herbs that can help with hot flashes and night sweats include anise, fennel, and sage.

Menstrual Cycle

From puberty to menopause, the menstrual cycle is a sign that a woman's body is going through the normal process of preparing for pregnancy. Although the length of the cycle varies from woman to woman, it is generally between twenty-one and thirty-five days.

Leukorrhea

A whitish or slightly yellowish discharge is a normal function that aids in keeping vaginal tissue healthy. Its characteristics may fluctuate over the course of the monthly cycle; however, if the discharge becomes excessive, extremely thick, or develops an unpleasant odor, it can be a sign of infection. These symptoms may be accompanied by itchiness, irritation, and pain. While leukorrhea can be caused by douching and using scented sprays, it is important to consult your doctor for a correct diagnosis. Leukorrhea can be indicative of a bacterial or yeast infection (*Candida albicans*), improper hygiene, or a sexually transmitted disease. In the past, leukorrhea was known as the whites.

❁ Aloe and Turmeric Gel

6 tablespoons aloe vera gel
2 teaspoons turmeric, powdered

Combine the aloe vera and turmeric and gently stir until thoroughly mixed. Store in a glass jar with a tight-fitting lid.

> ***To use:*** Apply to itchy or irritated areas several times a day or as needed. Because turmeric can stain clothing, you may want to wear a panty liner or pad.

❁ Basil and Yarrow Sitz Bath Infusion

1 cup dried basil, crumbled
1 cup dried yarrow, crumbled

1 cup baking soda (optional)
3 quarts water

Bring the water to a boil in a large stockpot, and then turn off the heat. Place the basil and yarrow in a muslin bag and add it to the water. Cover and steep for 2 hours.

> ***To use:*** Warm the infusion to a comfortable temperature, and then add it along with the bag of herbs and baking soda to shallow bathwater. Soak until the water begins to cool.

The astringent and anti-inflammatory properties of the ingredients used in these preparations help soothe the itching and other discomforts. Sage can also be used to ease leukorrhea. It helps to wear cotton underwear to avoid irritation from synthetic fabrics and to bathe with mild, nonallergenic soap.

Menstrual Cramps

Known medically as dysmenorrhea, menstrual cramps are caused by uterine contractions that occur when the lining of the uterus is not needed for pregnancy and is expelled. The resulting cramps can range from annoying to severe.

❁ Anise and Black Cohosh Tea

1 teaspoon aniseeds, crushed
1 teaspoon dried black cohosh, finely chopped
1 cup water, boiled

Lightly toast the aniseeds in a dry frying pan over low heat before crushing. Pre-warm a cup or mug with hot tap water, and then add the seeds, black cohosh, and boiled water. Cover and steep for 10 to 15 minutes before straining.

> ***To use:*** Warm, add a little honey to sweeten, and drink while comfortably hot. Take 2 to 3 cups a day.

❁ Feverfew and Lavender Tea

1 teaspoon dried feverfew, crumbled
1 teaspoon dried lavender, crumbled
1 cup water, boiled

Pre-warm a cup or mug with hot tap water, and then add the feverfew, lavender, and boiled water. Cover and steep for 10 to 15 minutes before straining.

> ***To use:*** Warm, add a little honey to sweeten, and drink while comfortably hot. Take 2 to 3 cups a day.

The antispasmodic properties of all these herbs help relieve menstrual cramps. Because thyme contains a number of minerals including iron, it is especially beneficial at the end of a menstrual period. With its antispasmodic and diuretic properties, angelica root eases cramps and helps relieve water retention. Other herbs to use for easing menstrual cramps include caraway, chamomile, coriander, dill, fennel, ginger, hyssop, lemon balm, oregano, parsley, peppermint, rosemary, St. John's wort, thyme, valerian, and yarrow. Resting with a heating pad or a warm compress on the abdomen also helps.

Premenstrual Syndrome (PMS)

PMS has a wide range of symptoms that include mood swings, irritability, depression, nervous tension, sleep problems, and lack of concentration. Physical symptoms include tender breasts, headache, fatigue, muscle aches, joint pain, abdominal bloating, and acne. While symptoms may occur in a predictable cycle, they can change in intensity from time to time.

❁ Lemon Balm, Nettle, and Thyme Infusion

3 tablespoons dried lemon balm, crumbled
2 tablespoons dried nettle, crumbled
1 tablespoon dried thyme, crumbled
1 quart water, boiled

Pre-warm a large jar with hot tap water, and then add the lemon balm, nettle, thyme, and boiled water. Cover and steep for 45 minutes before straining. Store in the refrigerator.

To use: Warm and drink a cup at a time. Take 2 to 3 cups a day while symptoms last.

❁ Dandelion and Ginger Decoction

3 tablespoons dried dandelion root, chopped
2 tablespoons dried ginger, chopped
1 quart water

Place the dandelion, ginger, and water in a saucepan and bring to a boil. Stir, cover, and reduce the heat to as low as possible. Simmer for 40 minutes, and then allow it to cool completely before straining. Store in the refrigerator.

To use: Warm and drink a cup at a time. Take 2 to 3 cups a day while symptoms last.

Lemon balm is an uplifting herb that soothes tension, stress, and moods. Thyme helps with headaches and muscle aches. Dandelion and ginger alleviate premenstrual bloating and other discomforts; ginger also helps with stress and moods. Fennel aids with a range of symptoms and helps reduce fluid retention. Black cohosh is effective for hormone-related headaches and migraines. Other herbs that ease PMS symptoms include chamomile, parsley, and St. John's wort.

Other steps to take when dealing with PMS are to avoid eating foods with high amounts of refined sugars, to get adequate sleep, and to exercise regularly. Just taking a walk every day can be especially helpful.

Prostatitis

Prostatitis is the inflammation and swelling of the prostate gland. Symptoms include discomfort or pain in the genitals and groin area, difficulty urinating, frequent or painful urination, flu-like symptoms, low back pain, and pain with ejaculation. While it is important to see your doctor for diagnosis and treatment, home remedies can help alleviate the discomfort.

❁ Burdock Sitz Bath Infusion

3 cups dried burdock root, finely chopped
4–5 quarts water

Bring the water to a boil in a large stockpot. Place the burdock in a muslin bag, add it to the water, and cover. Reduce the heat to as low as possible and simmer for 20 minutes. Turn off the heat and steep for 2 to 3 hours.

> ***To use:*** Warm to a comfortable temperature, and then add the infusion and bag of herbs to shallow bathwater. Soak until the water begins to cool.

❁ Nettle Compress

6 tablespoons dried nettle root, chopped
4 tablespoons dried nettle leaves, crumbled
1 quart water

Place the nettle root and water in a saucepan and bring to a boil. Stir, cover, and reduce the heat to as low as possible. Simmer for 30 minutes. Remove from the heat and add the nettle leaves. Cover and steep for 2 hours before straining.

> ***To use:*** Warm to a comfortable temperature. Soak and wring out a washcloth, and then place it over the perineal area. Apply for 15 to 20 minutes, freshening the cloth every 5 minutes or so.

The anti-inflammatory and diuretic properties of burdock and nettle have long been used for a range of problems relating to the urinary tract and prostate. A ½-cup dose of turmeric decoction taken twice a day is another remedy that helps ease the discomfort. All three of these herbs support a healthy prostate. Regular exercise is also helpful.

Vaginitis

Vaginitis is the infection or inflammation of vaginal tissue that can be caused by bacteria, a yeast infection, or a sexually transmitted disease (STD). Symptoms include a change in vaginal discharge, itching, and painful urination. It is important to catch a yeast infection in its early stages for home treatment to be effective.

❁ Garlic Treatment

1 teaspoon garlic juice
2 tablespoons yogurt

Using a garlic press, squeeze the juice out of several cloves and mix well with the yogurt.

> ***To use:*** Soak a tampon in the mixture before inserting. Leave overnight. Do this each night while symptoms last.

❁ Lavender and Sage Sitz Bath Infusion

2 cups dried lavender, crumbled
2 cups dried sage, crumbled
4–5 quarts water

Place the lavender and sage in a muslin bag and set aside. Bring the water to a boil in a large stockpot, turn off the heat, and add the bag of herbs. Cover and steep for 2 to 3 hours.

> ***To use:*** Warm to a comfortable temperature, and then add the infusion and bag of herbs to shallow bathwater. Soak until the water begins to cool.

The yogurt in the garlic treatment acts as a soothing medium to avoid burns that can occur when garlic juice is used directly on the skin. Garlic is not the most pleasant treatment, but it is effective. Bay laurel and lemongrass can also be used for vaginitis.

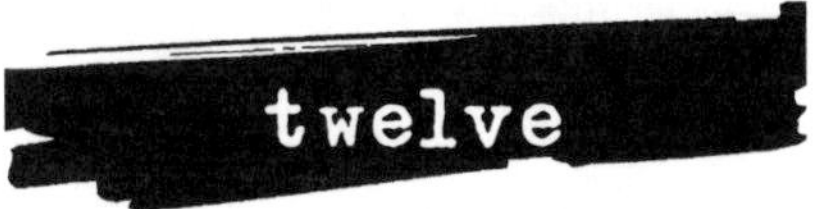

The Circulatory, Endocrine, and Urinary Systems

The circulatory system consists of a network of organs and blood vessels that carries oxygen, hormones, and nutrients to every cell in the body. It also carries waste away from the cells. The urinary system filters the blood and eliminates waste from the body. The endocrine system is a network of glands that regulates the body's functions.

The Circulatory and Lymphatic Systems

Consisting of the heart, veins, arteries, and capillaries, the circulatory system is instrumental in maintaining a stable environment within the body and fighting disease. Also known as the cardiovascular system, it has a pulmonary loop through the lungs to oxygenate the blood and release carbon dioxide, a waste product of the cells. Working in conjunction to remove bacteria and waste from the body, a subsystem called *the lymphatic system* produces lymph, a fluid that bathes the tissues and maintains the balance of fluids in the body. The lymphatic system includes the lymph nodes, spleen, tonsils, and adenoids, and produces white blood cells that protect the body against infection.

Chilblains

Chilblains are the painful inflammation of small blood vessels in the skin that appear a day or two after prolonged exposure to cold. Also known as pernio and chill burns, chilblains occur on the toes, hands, feet, ears, nose, and fingers. Unlike frostbite, it does not cause permanent damage. Symptoms can sometimes be intense and include itching or burning, dryness, swelling, redness, and blisters.

❁ Spearmint and Aloe Gel

For the infused oil:
2 tablespoons dried spearmint, crumbled
⅓ cup olive oil

For the gel:
3–4 tablespoons aloe vera gel
¼ cup infused oil

Place the spearmint and olive oil in a double boiler and cover. With the heat as low as possible, warm for 30 minutes. Remove from the heat and allow it to cool to room temperature before straining. Place the aloe gel in a bowl. Slowly add the infused oil until the gel reaches a consistency you like. Stir until it is thoroughly mixed. Store in a glass jar with a tight-fitting lid.

To use: Without rubbing, gently apply to affected areas.

❁ Ginger Salve

For the infused oil:
4 tablespoons fresh ginger, coarsely grated
⅔ cup jojoba oil

For the salve:
½ ounce beeswax, chopped into small pieces
8–9 tablespoons infused oil

Place the ginger in a small muslin bag in a double boiler. Add the jojoba oil and cover. With the heat as low as possible, warm for 30 minutes. Remove from the heat and allow the infused oil to cool slightly. Squeeze excess oil from the muslin bag. Combine the beeswax and infused oil in a glass jar and place it in a saucepan of water. Warm over low heat, stirring until the beeswax melts. Remove from the heat and allow the mixture to cool slightly. Test the consistency and adjust if necessary. Let it cool completely before using or storing.

To use: Without rubbing, gently apply to affected areas.

The anti-inflammatory properties of the ingredients in the salve and gel soothe and heal the skin. Both spearmint and ginger warm the skin; ginger also aids circulation. Avoid scratching chilblains as blisters may break open and become infected. Cayenne-infused oil can be used to treat chilblains but only if the blisters are not broken. Use ¼ teaspoon of powdered cayenne in 2 tablespoons of olive oil. Test on a small area of skin to make sure it does not feel too warm.

Edema and Lymphedema

Although edema and lymphedema are different ailments, their treatment is the same. Edema is the swelling that occurs when excess fluid from the capillaries builds up in the surrounding tissue. Some of the causes include sitting or standing in one place for too long, the weakening of the valves in the veins, some medications, allergies, and certain diseases. It can occur anywhere but most often occurs in the ankles, feet, legs, hands, and arms.

Lymphedema is the swelling caused by the inability of lymph fluid to flow properly through the lymph vessels and into the bloodstream. It usually occurs in one arm or leg, but sometimes both. It is often caused by a blockage in the lymph system or a problem with lymph nodes that prevents the normal drainage of lymph. While mild cases of edema and lymphedema usually go away on their own, it is best to consult with your doctor when any type of persistent swelling occurs.

❁Dandelion Massage Oil

¾ cup fresh dandelion root, chopped
1 cup coconut oil

Place the dandelion in a muslin bag in a double boiler. Add the coconut oil and cover. With the heat as low as possible, warm for 40 minutes. Allow the oil to cool completely, and then squeeze excess oil from the muslin bag.

To use: Place a little of the infused oil on your fingertips and gently but firmly massage the affected area using long strokes toward the heart.

❁ Angelica and Burdock Decoction

3 tablespoons dried angelica root, chopped
3 tablespoons dried burdock root, chopped
1 quart water

Place the angelica, burdock, and water in a saucepan and bring to a boil. Stir, cover, and reduce the heat to as low as possible. Simmer for 30 minutes, and then allow it to cool before straining. Store in the refrigerator.

To use: Warm and drink a cup at a time. Take 3 to 4 cups a day for 2 to 3 days.

Tea made with 2 teaspoons of coriander seeds or fennel seeds also helps reduce the swelling of edema and lymphedema. Ginger tea helps increase circulation and reduce inflammation. Consider using a combination of herbal tea, massage, exercise, and compression garments.

Swollen Glands/Lymph Nodes

Commonly referred to as lymph glands, lymph nodes help fight off infection by filtering lymphatic fluid and trapping bacteria or viruses before they can reach other parts of the body. Known medically as lymphadenitis, swollen lymph nodes are a sign that your body is dealing with an infection. Although lymph nodes are scattered throughout the body, the most common and noticeable swelling occurs in the neck, under the chin, armpits, and groin. Characterized by tenderness and sometimes pain, the swelling usually goes away on its own.

When accompanied by a sore throat, fever, or runny nose, swollen glands are an indication of a respiratory infection or a cold. It can also occur with strep throat, mononucleosis, and ear infection. In addition to easing the discomfort of swollen lymph nodes, it is important to treat the underlying condition. If swelling persists or occurs throughout the body, it may indicate other infections and you should consult your doctor.

❁ Chamomile and Peppermint Infusion

4 tablespoons dried chamomile, crumbled
2 tablespoons dried peppermint, crumbled
1 quart water, boiled

Pre-warm a large glass jar with hot tap water, and then add the chamomile, peppermint, and boiled water. Cover and steep for 40 minutes before straining. Store in the refrigerator.

To use: Warm and drink a cup at a time. Take up to 3 cups a day.

❁ Mullein and Sage Compress

6 tablespoons dried mullein root, chopped
4 tablespoons dried sage, crumbled
1 quart water

Place the mullein and water in a saucepan and bring to a boil. Stir, cover, and reduce the heat to as low as possible. Simmer for 20 minutes. Remove from the heat and add the sage. Cover and steep for 40 minutes before straining.

To use: Warm to a comfortable temperature. Soak and wring out a washcloth, and then place it over the swollen lymph nodes. Apply for 15 to 20 minutes, freshening the cloth every 5 minutes or so.

The anti-inflammatory, antibacterial, and antiviral properties of these herbs help deal with the swelling and fight infection. Adding garlic to your diet also helps fight infection, as does turmeric. Add 1 tablespoon of turmeric to a cup of warm milk and drink once a day. Other herbs to use for swollen lymph nodes include ginger, rosemary, and thyme.

Tonsillitis

Tonsillitis is an infection and inflammation of the tonsils that can be caused by bacteria or a virus. In addition to swollen tonsils, other symptoms include a sore throat and difficulty swallowing. The lymph nodes on the sides of the neck may be tender. While tonsillitis needs to be treated by a physician, herbal remedies as part of home care help fight infection and relieve the symptoms.

❁ Hyssop and Mullein Gargle

1 teaspoon dried hyssop, crumbled
1 teaspoon dried mullein, crumbled
¾ teaspoon table salt
1 cup water, boiled

Pre-warm a cup or mug with hot tap water before adding the hyssop, mullein, salt, and boiled water. Cover and steep for 15 minutes, and then strain.

To use: Warm to a comfortable temperature, and then gargle with a little at a time until it is gone. Gargle 2 to 3 times a day or as needed. A little lemon juice can be added, which will also help soothe the throat.

❁ Ginger and Chamomile Decoction

2 tablespoons fresh ginger, coarsely grated
4 tablespoons dried chamomile, crumbled
3 cups water

Place the ginger and water in a saucepan and bring to a boil. Stir, cover, and reduce the heat to as low as possible. Simmer for 30 minutes, and then remove from the heat and add the chamomile. Cover and steep for 15 minutes before straining. Store in the refrigerator.

To use: Warm and drink a cup at a time. Add honey if desired. Take 2 to 3 cups a day.

The antibacterial, antiviral, and anti-inflammatory properties of hyssop, mullein, ginger, and chamomile soothe inflamed tonsils and help fight infection. The Garlic Syrup included under Sinusitis in Chapter 6 is also effective. Other herbs to use for tonsillitis include burdock, lavender, oregano, peppermint, sage, and thyme.

Varicose Veins

Varicose veins are enlarged veins close to the skin surface that usually appear dark blue and gnarled. They are sometimes accompanied by swelling. For some, they can be painful with a burning or throbbing sensation. Varicose veins most often occur in the legs because of increased pressure due to excessive standing. They can be exacerbated by pregnancy and overweight. Occurring in the capillaries, spider veins are a mild variation of varicose veins.

❁ Yarrow Liniment

6 tablespoons dried yarrow, crumbled
2 cups witch hazel

Place the yarrow and witch hazel in a glass jar with a tight-fitting lid. Close and shake for 1 or 2 minutes. Set aside for 4 to 6 weeks, giving the jar a good shake every day. Strain before using.

> ***To use:*** Twice a day, gently rub a little of the liniment on the area around the veins in an upward motion toward the heart. Do not rub the veins directly.

❁ St. John's Wort and Rosemary Fomentation

For the cool compress:
10 tablespoons dried St. John's wort, crumbled
1 quart water

For the warm compress:
10 tablespoons dried rosemary, crumbled
1 quart water

A fomentation is the process of alternating warm and cool compresses. Make the cool compress infusion first to give it time to chill. Pre-warm a large glass jar, and then add the St. John's wort and boiled water. Cover and steep for 45 minutes before straining. Place it in the refrigerator to chill. Follow the same steps using rosemary to make the warm compress. Strain and let it cool to a comfortable temperature.

> ***To use:*** Soak and wring out a washcloth in the rosemary (warm) infusion, and then place it over the affected area. Freshen the cloth every 5 minutes or so for 15 minutes. Use the St. John's wort (cool) infusion the same way. Repeat the process of applying the warm and then the cool compress 2 more times, warming or chilling the infusions as needed. Apply the fomentation twice a day.

Yarrow, rosemary, and St. John's wort help reduce swelling; witch hazel helps tone and tighten the skin. Instead of a liniment, use an infused oil to gently massage the area around the veins in an upward motion toward the heart. Drinking St. John's wort tea helps relieve varicose veins, too. Physical exercise, elevating the legs while resting, and avoiding long periods of sitting also help.

The Endocrine System

The endocrine system consists of a network of glands that produce and secrete hormones to regulate various body functions such as growth and development, reproduction, and tissue function. Some of the glands in the endocrine system include the pineal, thyroid, thymus, adrenals, testes, and ovaries.

Goiter

Goiter is the enlargement of the thyroid, a butterfly-shaped gland at the base of the neck just below the Adam's apple. The thyroid produces hormones that regulate the body's metabolism. Goiter is characterized by swelling around the front of the neck and sometimes a tight sensation in the throat. Although it is most commonly due to iodine deficiency, goiter can be caused by inflammation or other conditions that your doctor needs to diagnose, especially if you have difficulty swallowing or breathing. Although iodine can be added to the diet with iodized salt, foods such as seafood, seaweed, watercress, and others are a healthier source.

❁ Nettle and Lemon Balm Tea

1 teaspoon dried nettle, crumbled
1 teaspoon dried lemon balm, crumbled
1 cup water, boiled

Pre-warm a cup or mug with hot tap water, and then add the nettle, lemon balm, and boiled water. Cover and steep for 10 to 15 minutes before straining.

To use: Warm and drink while it is comfortably hot. Take 2 to 3 cups a day.

❁ Dandelion and Parsley Poultice

2 tablespoons dried dandelion, crumbled
2 tablespoons dried parsley, crumbled
2–3 cups water

Place the dandelion and parsley in a muslin bag and set aside. Bring the water to a boil in a saucepan, and then remove it from the heat. Place the bag of herbs in the water for 2 to 3 minutes to moisten and warm them. Remove from the water and press out excess moisture.

> ***To use:*** Check that the bag of herbs is not too hot, and then set it directly on the affected area. Cover the poultice with a towel to keep it warm for as long as possible. Remove when it starts to cool. Apply a poultice 2 or 3 times a day, making it fresh each time.

Adding garlic to your diet also helps reduce goiter development. Lemon balm and garlic aid in healthy thyroid function. Nettle is a nutritive herb and a source of iodine. Dandelion and parsley also work well to drink as tea because of their cleansing properties.

The Urinary System

Also known as the urinary tract and renal system, its function is to remove waste from the body. Urine is created by the kidneys as they filter the blood, removing waste and extra water. The kidneys keep water and chemicals, such as sodium, in balance and help regulate blood pressure. The bladder stores urine and controls its release.

Bladder Infection

Cystitis, or inflammation of the bladder, is caused by a bacterial infection. It is the most common type of urinary tract infection (UTI). Symptoms may include the frequent urge to urinate, pain or a burning sensation while urinating, cloudy or bloody urine, lower abdominal pain, and low back pain.

Fever and chills may also occur. While is it important to consult with your doctor, home care treatments can aid recovery.

❁ Nettle, Dandelion, and Angelica Decoction

3 tablespoons fresh nettle root, chopped
2 tablespoons fresh dandelion root, chopped
2 tablespoons fresh angelica root, chopped
1 quart water

Place the nettle, dandelion, angelica, and water in a saucepan and bring to a boil. Stir, cover, and reduce the heat to as low as possible. Simmer for 25 to 30 minutes, and then allow it to cool completely before straining. Store in the refrigerator.

> ***To use:*** Warm and drink a cup at a time. Take 2 to 3 cups a day.

❁ Mullein and Yarrow Compress

6 tablespoons dried mullein, crumbled
4 tablespoons dried yarrow, crumbled
1 quart water

Pre-warm a large glass jar, and then add the mullein, yarrow, and boiled water. Cover and steep for 1 hour before straining.

> ***To use:*** Warm to a comfortable temperature. Soak and wring out a washcloth, and then place it over the pubic area. Apply for 15 to 20 minutes, freshening the cloth every 5 minutes or so.

Nettle root helps increase urine production and its astringent properties help soothe inflammation of the urinary tract. In addition to its diuretic properties, dandelion root is a restorative herb for the urinary tract. Angelica is a diuretic that helps tone the urinary system. A warm sitz bath can also help alleviate pain. Other herbs for soothing bladder infection and inflammation include burdock, garlic, ginger, parsley, and St. John's wort.

While dealing with a bladder infection, women should avoid products that contain fragrance oils such as tampons, sanitary pads, douches, sprays, and bubble bath. It also helps to drink plenty of water to flush out bacteria.

Kidney Stones

Minerals and salts occasionally build up in the kidneys and produce hard deposits. They may not cause trouble and even remain unknown until they pass into the ureter, the narrow tube that connects the kidney to the bladder. Pain can be severe and occur on one side on the back or the lower abdomen. Other symptoms may include pink, red, or brown urine, painful urination, nausea, and vomiting. There is no single cause for kidney stones; however, contributing factors include diet, dehydration, obesity, family history, and some medical conditions.

❁ Fennel and Basil Tea

1 teaspoon fennel seeds, crushed
1 teaspoon dried basil, crumbled
1 cup water, boiled

Lightly toast the fennel seeds in a dry frying pan over low heat before crushing. Pre-warm a cup or mug with hot tap water, and then add the fennel seeds, basil, and boiled water. Cover and steep for 10 to 15 minutes before straining.

To use: Drink 2 to 3 cups a day.

❁ Mullein and Nettle Poultice

2 tablespoons dried mullein leaves, crumbled
2 tablespoons dried nettle leaves, crumbled
2 cups water

Place the mullein and nettle in a muslin bag and set aside. Bring the water to a boil in a saucepan, and then remove it from the heat. Place the bag of herbs in the water for 1 to 3 minutes to moisten and warm them. Remove from the water and press out excess moisture.

To use: While comfortably warm, place the bag of herbs over the painful area and cover with a towel to keep the poultice warm for as long as possible. Remove when it starts to cool. Apply a poultice 2 or 3 times a day, making it fresh each time.

Fennel is a diuretic, and basil contains components that can aid in dissolving a kidney stone. If you have a juicer, use a handful of fresh basil leaves blended with a stalk or two of celery to help flush out the stone. Parsley can also be used as tea. In addition to being diuretics that can be used internally, mullein and fennel have anti-inflammatory and antispasmodic properties that make them topically effective, too.

Instead of a poultice, they can be used to make an infusion and applied as a warm compress. A fomentation alternating warm and cool compresses can also help. As with bladder infections, drink plenty of water.

thirteen

Common Kitchen Herbs and Spices

While herbs are often regarded simply as seasoning, most of them have been used medicinally for centuries. This chapter will help you become familiar with the medicinal properties of the common kitchen and tea herbs included this book. Also contained in the following entries are plant descriptions, botanical names, medicinal properties, and precautions and contraindications.

Anise

Spicy, sweet, and licorice-like, anise may be a familiar taste in commercial cough syrups and lozenges, but this herb can do more than add flavor. Long used to settle digestive upsets, its estrogen-like properties also soothe menstrual cramps and menopausal discomforts.

Only reaching about two feet tall, anise looks like a small, spindly version of Queen Anne's lace. Its lower leaves are rounded; the upper leaves are feathery. Umbels of delicate yellowish-white flowers grow at the tops of the stems.

Botanical names: Pimpinella anisum, syn. *Anisum officinalis, A. vulgare*

Also known as: Aniseed, sweet cumin, pimpinel seed

Parts used: Mostly the seeds; sometimes the leaves

Precautions and contraindications: Avoid during pregnancy; do not use when taking medication that clots the blood; should not be used by anyone with a condition that may worsen by exposure to estrogen. Do not confuse with star anise (*Illicium verum*)

Medicinal properties: Antibacterial, antimicrobial, antiseptic, antispasmodic, antiviral, estrogenic, expectorant, stimulant

Used for: Asthma, bloating, breastfeeding, bronchitis, common cold, congestion, cough, fever, flatulence, flu, halitosis, head lice, hot flashes and night sweats, indigestion, insomnia and sleep, menopausal discomforts, menstrual cramps, nausea, postpartum blues, scabies, shin splints, sinusitis, stomach pain, stress and anxiety

Basil

Perhaps best known for its flavor in pesto and pasta sauce, basil also helps fight infection. In addition to supporting a healthy digestive system, its soothing qualities can ease anxiety and stress. Not only does it relieve insect bites, basil can also be used to repel bugs.

Basil is a bushy plant that reaches one to two feet tall. Its oval leaves have prominent veins and a distinctive downward curl. They are yellow-green to dark green and very fragrant. Blooming from midsummer to autumn, clusters of white, pink, or purple flowers grow on separate flower spikes.

Botanical name: Ocimum basilicum
Also known as: Common basil, French basil, sweet basil
Parts used: Leaves
Precautions and contraindications: Therapeutic doses should be avoided during pregnancy and while breastfeeding
Medicinal properties: Antibacterial, anti-inflammatory, antispasmodic, antiviral, astringent, sedative
Used for: Bronchitis, canker sores, common cold, constipation, cough, flatulence, flu, gingivitis, halitosis, headache, indigestion, insect bites and beestings, insomnia and sleep, kidney stones, mental fatigue, motion sickness, nausea, nervous tension, sinusitis, stomach pain, stress and anxiety, warts

Bay Laurel

Best known for its spicy aroma and earthy taste, bay provides flavorful depth to soups, stews, and many other dishes. For the medicine cabinet, its various properties make it a good choice for a wide range of ailments.

Although this evergreen tree can grow up to fifty feet tall, it is usually kept pruned as a shrub. The leathery, dark green leaves are oval and sharply pointed. Bay has greenish-yellow flowers that grow in tiny clusters. Its small oval berries turn bluish-black when ripe.

Botanical name: Laurus nobilis
Also known as: Bay, bay tree, sweet bay, true laurel
Parts used: Leaves

Precautions and contraindications: Do not use bay laurel when taking pain or sedative medications; avoid during pregnancy and while breastfeeding

Medicinal properties: Analgesic, antibacterial, antifungal, anti-inflammatory, antiviral, astringent, diuretic, expectorant, nervine

Used for: Arthritis, asthma, athlete's foot, bloating, bruises, carpal tunnel syndrome, common cold, congestion, dandruff, flatulence, flu, indigestion, insect bites and beestings, jock itch, muscle soreness and stiffness, scabies, sciatica, sinusitis, sore throat, sprains and strains, vaginitis

Caraway

Caraway is most widely known for its flavorful seeds, which are popularly used to enhance breads, cakes, cheeses, and other foods. Long used as an aid to the digestive system, caraway seeds are a powerhouse when it comes to treating other ailments, too.

Reaching eighteen to twenty-four inches tall, caraway has feathery, light green leaves and tiny white flowers that grow in umbel clusters. They bloom in late summer. The slightly crescent-shaped seeds are ridged and pointed at both ends. Caraway is closely related to anise, dill, and fennel.

Botanical name: Carum carvi

Also known as: Common caraway, Roman cumin

Parts used: Mostly the seeds, sometimes the leaves

Precautions and contraindications: Excessive amounts of seeds should not be eaten during pregnancy

Medicinal properties: Analgesic, anti-inflammatory, antispasmodic, diuretic, expectorant

Used for: Belching, bloating, breastfeeding, bronchitis, bruises, colic, congestion, cough, flatulence, halitosis, heartburn/GERD, indigestion, irritable bowel syndrome (IBS), menstrual cramps, postpartum blues, stomach pain

Cayenne

In addition to adding a kick to food, cayenne is beneficial for the heart and cardiovascular health. It stimulates blood circulation and supports the immune system. Externally, cayenne is warming and soothing for a range of issues.

Reaching two to three feet tall, cayenne has broad, dark green leaves and white to yellowish-white flowers that grow in drooping pairs or clusters. The long, thin peppers start out green, then turn various shades of red, orange, or yellow as they ripen.

Botanical name: Capsicum annuum

Also known as: Capsicum, chili pepper, red chilies

Parts used: Fruit/peppers

Precautions and contraindications: Use in small amounts and in moderation; excessive internal use may cause upset stomach and kidney damage; those with irritable bowel syndrome (IBS) or chronic bowel inflammation should avoid the internal use of cayenne; may aggravate acidity and heartburn; may increase hot flashes during menopause; prolonged application to the skin may cause dermatitis

Medicinal properties: analgesic, anesthetic, antibacterial, anti-inflammatory, antimicrobial, antispasmodic, antioxidant, stimulant

Used for: Arthritis, bursitis and tendonitis, carpal tunnel syndrome, chilblains, common cold, congestion, cuts and abrasions, diarrhea, flatulence, flu, gout, hangover, headache, low back pain, migraine, motion sickness, muscle soreness and stiffness, muscle spasm and cramp, nerve pain, rheumatoid arthritis, sciatica, shin splints, shingles, sore throat, stomach pain

Chamomile, German

There are two types of chamomile; both have medicinal properties and, in many cases, can be used interchangeably. However, German chamomile has more medicinal properties that make it especially valuable for treating a wider range of problems.

With branching stems, German chamomile can reach two to three feet tall. It has feathery leaves and small, daisy-like flowers with white petals and yellow centers.

Botanical names: Matricaria recutita, syn. *M. chamomilla, Chamomilla chamomilla*

Also known as: Mayweed, wild chamomile

Parts used: Flowers

Precautions and contraindications: Although chamomile is an antiallergenic for most people, those who have allergies to plants in the Asteraceae/Compositae (aster/daisy) family should check for sensitivity before using it; avoid ingesting when taking prescription blood thinners

Medicinal properties: Antiallergenic, antibacterial, antifungal, antihistamine, anti-inflammatory, antioxidant, antiseptic, antispasmodic, antiviral, nervine

Used for: Acne, arthritis, asthma, belching, bloating, burns and scalds, canker sores, carpal tunnel syndrome, colic, common cold, cuts and abrasions, dandruff, dermatitis, earache, eczema, eyes (puffy), fever, flatulence, hay fever, headache, heartburn/GERD, hemorrhoids, hives, indigestion, insect bites and beestings, insomnia and sleep, irritable bowel syndrome (IBS), jock itch, laryngitis, mastitis, menopausal discomforts, menstrual cramps, motion sickness, muscle soreness and stiffness, muscle spasm and cramp, nausea, nerve pain, nervous tension, postpartum blues, premenstrual syndrome (PMS), psoriasis, rheumatoid arthritis, sciatica, shin splints, sore throat, sprains and strains, stomach pain, stress and anxiety, sties and chalazia, sunburn, swollen glands/lymph nodes, tonsillitis, toothache

Coriander

The sweet, slightly spicy seeds of coriander are used worldwide for culinary and medicinal purposes. For centuries, coriander has been used to settle digestive problems and to soothe pain. Known as cilantro, the lower leaves are popular in a range of dishes and sometimes used medicinally.

Growing one to two feet tall, the lower leaves (cilantro) are rounded; the upper leaves are feathery. Clusters of tiny white to pale lilac or mauve flowers bloom from summer to early autumn. The round seeds have a musty odor that changes to warm and spicy as they ripen.

Botanical name: Coriandrum sativum
Also known as: Chinese parsley (cilantro), coriander seed
Parts used: Mostly the seeds; sometimes the leaves
Precautions and contraindications: Those who are allergic to aniseed, caraway, fennel, or dill may have a reaction to this plant
Medicinal properties: analgesic, antibacterial, anti-inflammatory, antimicrobial, antispasmodic, nervine; leaves: antibacterial, anti-inflammatory, antispasmodic, astringent
Used for: Acne, arthritis, bloating, bronchitis, canker sores, cough, diarrhea, edema and lymphedema, fever, flatulence, halitosis, headache, heartburn/GERD, hemorrhoids, indigestion, insomnia and sleep, menstrual cramps, mental fatigue, muscle soreness and stiffness, muscle spasm and cramp, nausea, nerve pain, nervous tension, stomach pain, stress and anxiety, sties and chalazia, temporomandibular joint (TMJ) pain

Dill

Most famously known for adding a tang to pickles, dill's pungent seeds and flavorful leaves have wide culinary use. Dill contains a number of vitamins and minerals that support a healthy digestive system.

Reaching up to three feet tall, dill has ferny, blue-green leaves and large, flat umbel clusters of yellow flowers. Its oval seeds are flat and ribbed. Dill is closely related to anise, caraway, and fennel.

Botanical name: Anethum graveolens
Also known as: Dill weed (dried leaves), dillseed, dilly, garden dill
Parts used: Leaves, seeds
Precautions and contraindications: Avoid in medicinal concentrations during pregnancy; dill pickles are okay
Medicinal properties: analgesic, antibacterial, anti-inflammatory, antispasmodic, diuretic, expectorant, sedative
Used for: Arthritis, asthma, breastfeeding, bronchitis, colic, common cold, congestion, constipation, cough, flatulence, halitosis, headache, heartburn/GERD, hemorrhoids, indigestion, insomnia and sleep, menstrual cramps, nervous tension, postpartum blues, stomach pain

Fennel

Fennel's anise-like flavor makes it easy to work into a range of dishes. A calming medicinal herb, fennel helps heal and keep the digestive system healthy. Among its many medicinal uses, fennel is especially toning for the female reproductive system.

Reaching four to five feet tall, fennel has a white bulbous base with multiple stalks. It has feathery leaves and tiny bright-yellow flowers that grow in large umbel clusters. Its flat, oval seeds are light brown and ridged. Fennel is a cousin to anise, caraway, and dill.

Botanical names: Foeniculum vulgare, syn. *F. officinale*
Also known as: Bitter fennel, common fennel, wild fennel
Parts used: Leaves, seeds

Precautions and contraindications: Avoid during pregnancy; avoid with epilepsy or other seizure disorders; use in moderation; should not be given to children under the age of six

Medicinal properties: Analgesic, anti-inflammatory, antispasmodic, diuretic, expectorant, stimulant

Used for: Asthma, belching, bloating, breastfeeding, bronchitis, bruises, colic, congestion, cough, edema and lymphedema, eyes (puffy), fever, flatulence, heartburn/GERD, hot flashes and night sweats, indigestion, insect bites and beestings, irritable bowel syndrome (IBS), kidney stones, laryngitis, menopausal discomforts, menstrual cramps, motion sickness, nausea, postpartum blues, premenstrual syndrome (PMS), sore throat, stomach pain

Garlic

The medicinal properties of garlic make it an excellent choice for treating a range of problems. Including it in the diet stimulates digestion, promotes cardiovascular health, and supports the immune system. Its infection-fighting power even extends to staph infections.

Reaching one to two feet tall, garlic has flat, pointed leaves growing from a single stem that sprouts from the bulb. The bulb contains four to fifteen cloves that are encased in white papery skin. Separate leafless stems produce globe-shaped clusters of small white to pinkish flowers.

Botanical name: Allium sativum

Also known as: Common garlic, stinking rose, stinkweed

Parts used: Bulb, separated into cloves

Precautions and contraindications: Large amounts may cause heartburn or irritate the stomach; avoid while breastfeeding; garlic applied directly to the skin may cause burns

Medicinal properties: Antibacterial, antifungal, antimicrobial, antiseptic, antispasmodic, antiviral, diuretic, expectorant

Used for: Athlete's foot, bladder infection, bronchitis, catarrh, common cold, congestion, cough, cuts and abrasions, earache, flu, goiter, irritable bowel syndrome (IBS), jock itch, ringworm, scabies, sinusitis, sore throat, swollen glands/lymph nodes, tonsillitis, vaginitis, warts

Ginger

Revered as a culinary spice for its pungent taste and aroma, ginger has been used medicinally since ancient times. It is rich in vitamins and minerals and aids digestion. Ginger is a tonic for the male and female reproductive systems.

Ginger is a tropical perennial that grows about three feet tall. Its lance-shaped leaves grow in two rows along stems that sprout from the rhizome. Greenish-yellow flowers grow on separate stems. The thick, branched rhizomes form gnarly clumps. Ginger is related to turmeric.

Botanical name: Zingiber officinale

Also known as: Common ginger, gingerroot, true ginger

Parts used: Root/rhizome

Precautions and contraindications: Avoid with blood-thinning medications; avoid medicinal amounts during pregnancy and while breastfeeding; do not take if you have gallstones

Medicinal properties: Analgesic, antibacterial, anti-inflammatory, antiseptic, antiviral, astringent, diuretic, expectorant

Used for: Arthritis, asthma, belching, bladder infection, bloating, bursitis and tendonitis, chilblains, cold sores, common cold, congestion, constipation, cough, cuts and abrasions, edema and lymphedema, fever, flatulence, flu, gout, hay fever, headache, heartburn/GERD, indigestion, low back pain, mastitis, menstrual cramps, mental fatigue, motion sickness, muscle soreness and stiffness, nausea, nerve pain, premenstrual syndrome (PMS), rheumatoid arthritis, sciatica, shin splints, sinusitis, sore throat, stress and anxiety, swollen glands/lymph nodes, tonsillitis, toothache

Lemon Balm

Lemon balm makes a delightful tea, but after a hectic day, it can seem almost magical as it calms the nerves and digestive system. Lemon balm has been cultivated as a medicinal herb for several thousand years. Its antioxidants help support and strengthen the immune system.

Reaching one to three feet tall, lemon balm is a bushy plant with deeply veined, bright-green leaves that have a noticeable lemony scent. Growing in clusters, the small white to yellowish flowers bloom from midsummer to early autumn.

Botanical name: Melissa officinalis

Also known as: Honey balm, melissa, sweet balm

Parts used: Leaves, stems

Precautions and contraindications: May interact with sedative and thyroid medications

Medicinal properties: Analgesic, antibacterial, antifungal, anti-inflammatory, antispasmodic, antiviral, sedative

Used for: Acne, asthma, bronchitis, cold sores, common cold, congestion, cough, dermatitis, eczema, fever, flatulence, flu, goiter, headache, heartburn/GERD, indigestion, insect bites and beestings, insomnia and sleep, irritable bowel syndrome (IBS), menopausal discomforts, menstrual cramps, migraine, nerve pain, nervous tension, postpartum blues, premenstrual syndrome (PMS), psoriasis, sciatica, seasonal affective disorder (SAD), shingles, sinusitis, stomach pain, stress and anxiety

Oregano

Best known for adding flavor to pizza and pasta sauce, oregano is high in several vitamins, iron, and calcium. Like other members of the mint family, oregano is an aid for digestive issues. It is closely related to marjoram and is often confused with it.

Oregano is a perennial that can reach almost three feet tall. It has squarish red stems and deeply veined oval leaves. Clusters of deep pink to purple flowers grow at the ends of the stems and in the leaf axils.

Botanical name: Origanum vulgare

Also known as: Mountain mint, wild marjoram, winter marjoram

Parts used: Leaves, flowers

Precautions and contraindications: Avoid medicinal doses during pregnancy and while breastfeeding

Medicinal properties: Antibacterial, antihistamine, anti-inflammatory, antiseptic, antispasmodic, expectorant, nervine

Used for: Asthma, bronchitis, catarrh, common cold, congestion, constipation, cough, cuts and abrasions, flatulence, flu, headache, indigestion, insomnia and sleep, menstrual cramps, migraine, motion sickness, muscle soreness and stiffness, nervous tension, sore throat, sprains and strains, temporomandibular joint (TMJ) pain, tonsillitis

Parsley

Often regarded as just a decorative garnish, this seemingly humble herb is a nutritional powerhouse. It is high in several vitamins, calcium, iron, and magnesium.

Growing in rounded mounds, parsley is a biennial that reaches about a foot tall. Tiny yellow-green flowers grow on separate stalks. The oval seeds are grayish-brown and ribbed. The white root looks like a small parsnip. There are two types of parsley that can be used interchangeably: flat-leaf and curly-leaf. The flat-leaf variety has a slightly stronger flavor.

Botanical names: Petroselinum crispum, syn. *P. sativum* (curly-leaf); *Petroselinum crispum* var. *neapolitanum* (flat-leaf)

Also known as: common parsley, garden parsley, rock parsley (curly-leaf); Italian parsley, plain-leaf parsley (flat-leaf)

Parts used: Leaves, roots, seeds

Precautions and contraindications: Excessive amounts of the seeds can be toxic; avoid during pregnancy and while breastfeeding; those with kidney disease should avoid

Medicinal properties: Antihistamine, antispasmodic, diuretic, expectorant

Used for: Arthritis, asthma, bladder infection, breastfeeding, bruises, constipation, cough, dandruff, eyes (puffy), flatulence, goiter, gout, halitosis, hay fever, head lice, headache, hives, insect bites and beestings, kidney stones, mastitis, menstrual cramps, premenstrual syndrome (PMS)

Peppermint

Widely used for confectionery and beverages, peppermint is known for calming digestive complaints. Balancing intestinal flora and reducing inflammation are a bonus to its popular flavor. Peppermint is also helpful for soothing the nerves.

Peppermint grows from two to three feet tall. Its dark green leaves are deeply veined. Blooming from midsummer to early autumn, tiny purple, pink, or white flowers grow in whorls at the tops of the stems.

Botanical name: Mentha x piperita
Also known as: Balm mint, brandy mint
Parts used: Mainly leaves; sometimes flowers
Precautions and contraindications: Avoid with high blood pressure; do not use when pregnant or while breastfeeding; not compatible with homeopathic treatments; use in moderation; do not give to children under the age of five; avoid with hiatal hernia and acute gallstones
Medicinal properties: Antibacterial, anti-inflammatory, antimicrobial, antiseptic, antispasmodic, antiviral, astringent, nervine
Used for: Acne, asthma, belching, bloating, bronchitis, burns and scalds, bursitis and tendonitis, common cold, congestion, cough, diarrhea, eczema, fever, flatulence, flu,

gingivitis, halitosis, headache, heartburn/GERD, indigestion, insect bites and beestings, insomnia and sleep, irritable bowel syndrome (IBS), laryngitis, menstrual cramps, mental fatigue, migraine, motion sickness, muscle soreness and stiffness, muscle spasm and cramp, nausea, nerve pain, nervous tension, sinusitis, sore throat, sprains and strains, stomach pain, sunburn, swollen glands/lymph nodes, tonsillitis, toothache

Rosemary

The resinous yet sweet flavor of rosemary has made it a versatile culinary herb. Used medicinally for several thousand years, this warming herb promotes blood circulation and supports the nervous system. Rosemary is also good for the immune system and digestive tract.

Rosemary is a shrubby evergreen that grows two to six feet tall. Mature stems are woody. It has short, stiff, needle-like leaves that are dark green on top and pale underneath. Pale blue flowers grow in small clusters along the branches with the leaves.

Botanical name: Rosmarinus officinalis
Also known as: Compass plant, garden rosemary, rosmarine
Parts used: Leaves, flowers
Precautions and contraindications: Avoid during pregnancy and while breastfeeding; avoid with high blood pressure and with epilepsy; too much may irritate the stomach

Medicinal properties: Analgesic, antibacterial, anti-inflammatory, antioxidant, antiseptic, antispasmodic, antiviral, astringent, expectorant, nervine

Used for: Acne, arthritis, asthma, bloating, bronchitis, bruises, bursitis and tendonitis, canker sores, common cold, congestion, cuts and abrasions, dandruff, eczema, eyes (puffy), flatulence, flu, halitosis, headache, hives, indigestion, irritable bowel syndrome (IBS), low back pain, menstrual cramps, mental fatigue, migraine, muscle soreness and stiffness, muscle spasm and cramp, nervous tension, sinusitis, sore throat, sprains and strains, stomach pain, stress and anxiety, sunburn, swollen glands/lymph nodes, temporomandibular joint (TMJ) pain, varicose veins

Sage

Don't wait until Thanksgiving to get sage out of the cupboard because cold and flu season starts in October and this herb can help soothe and prevent illness. Sage is a tonic for the nervous system and its estrogenic properties are helpful during menopause.

Sage grows one to three feet tall and has woody base stems. Its oblong leaves are grayish-green, wrinkled, and puckered. Leafy stalks bear whorls of small bluish-purple flowers that bloom early to midsummer.

Botanical name: Salvia officinalis

Also known as: Common sage, garden sage, true sage

Parts used: Leaves

Precautions and contraindications: Should not be used on a daily basis; use in moderation; avoid during pregnancy and while breastfeeding; avoid with epilepsy or other seizure disorder; avoid with high blood pressure and diabetes
Medicinal properties: Antibacterial, antifungal, anti-inflammatory, antiseptic, antiviral, astringent, estrogenic, nervine
Used for: Acne, arthritis, asthma, boils and carbuncles, breastfeeding, canker sores, carpal tunnel syndrome, catarrh, common cold, congestion, cuts and abrasions, dandruff, diarrhea, fever, flu, gingivitis, halitosis, headache, hemorrhoids, hot flashes and night sweats, insect bites and beestings, insomnia and sleep, laryngitis, menopausal discomforts, mental fatigue, muscle soreness and stiffness, nervous tension, sinusitis, sore throat, swollen glands/lymph nodes, tonsillitis, vaginitis

Spearmint

Although it is sweeter and milder than peppermint, spearmint is just as effective for many ailments and is better for treating children's ailments. Spearmint is an amphoteric herb that does what is needed; it can stimulate or relax, warm or cool.

Spearmint has tight whorls of pink or lilac flowers atop spikes of bright-green leaves. Like peppermint, its leaves are deeply veined. It reaches twelve to eighteen inches tall and blooms from late summer to early autumn.

Botanical names: Mentha spicata, syn. *M. viridis*
Also known as: Green mint, lamb mint, sage of Bethlehem
Parts used: Mainly leaves; sometimes flowers

Precautions and contraindications: Generally regarded as safe
Medicinal properties: analgesic, antibacterial, anti-inflammatory, antimicrobial, antispasmodic, astringent, diuretic
Used for: Acne, asthma, belching, bronchitis, burns and scalds, chilblains, colic, common cold, congestion, cough, fever, flatulence, gingivitis, halitosis, heartburn/GERD, hot flashes and night sweats, indigestion, insect bites and beestings, insomnia and sleep, laryngitis, low back pain, motion sickness, muscle soreness and stiffness, nausea, sore throat, stress and anxiety, sunburn, toothache

Thyme

For centuries, this popular seasoning was used as a food preservative. Thyme has been widely used for medicinal purposes, too. It fights infection and provides support for the immune, digestive, and nervous systems.

Reaching eight to twelve inches tall, thyme is a shrubby herb with woody base stems. The lance-shaped leaves are grayish-green on top and lighter underneath. Blooming in midsummer, the small pink to lilac or bluish-purple flowers grow in little clusters at the ends of the stems.

Botanical name: Thymus vulgaris
Also known as: Common thyme, English thyme, sweet thyme
Parts used: Leaves, flowers
Precautions and contraindications: Avoid during pregnancy and while breastfeeding; avoid with high blood pressure; do not use if you have a duodenal ulcer

Medicinal properties: Analgesic, antibacterial, antifungal, anti-inflammatory, antioxidant, antiseptic, antispasmodic, antiviral, expectorant, nervine

Used for: Acne, arthritis, asthma, athlete's foot, bloating, boils and carbuncles, bronchitis, bruises, canker sores, catarrh, common cold, congestion, cough, cuts and abrasions, diarrhea, earache, flatulence, flu, gingivitis, halitosis, hangover, hay fever, head lice, headache, indigestion, jock itch, laryngitis, low back pain, menopausal discomforts, menstrual cramps, migraine, muscle soreness and stiffness, muscle spasm and cramp, premenstrual syndrome (PMS), ringworm, scabies, sciatica, shin splints, sinusitis, sore throat, sprains and strains, stomach pain, sties and chalazia, swollen glands/lymph nodes, tonsillitis, toothache, warts

Turmeric

Turmeric is a warming spice that adds a golden color to curry and other foods. It has been used in Ayurvedic and traditional Chinese medicine for several thousand years. Rich in antioxidants, turmeric supports the immune system and is in clinical studies for reducing the risk of cancer, stroke, and heart attack.

Reaching three feet tall, turmeric's heavily veined leaves grow directly from the rhizome. Its yellowish-white flowers are tinged with pink or purple and grow on separate stalks. The cylindrical rhizome is gnarly and sometimes branched. Turmeric is a cousin to ginger.

Botanical names: Curcuma longa, syn. *C. domestica*

Also known as: Indian saffron, turmeric ginger

Parts used: Root/rhizome

Precautions and contraindications: Do not take medicinal amounts orally during pregnancy or while breastfeeding; avoid with gallstones and bile duct obstruction; avoid with blood-thinning medications; may temporarily stain the skin and clothing when used topically; do not use for long periods of time as it may cause stomach distress

Medicinal properties: Antibacterial, anti-inflammatory, antioxidant, antiseptic, antiviral, astringent

Used for: Arthritis, asthma, bursitis and tendonitis, carpal tunnel syndrome, cuts and abrasions, eczema, flatulence, gingivitis, gout, halitosis, headache, indigestion, low back pain, motion sickness, nausea, nerve pain, prostatitis, psoriasis, rheumatoid arthritis, ringworm, stomach pain, sties and chalazia, swollen glands/lymph nodes

fourteen

Additional Herbs and Other Ingredients

This chapter covers additional herbs mentioned throughout this book. Some of them are culinary herbs, some are decorative garden plants, and others are often regarded as weeds. Whether or not a plant is a weed or an herb is determined in the eye of the beholder. According to *Webster's* dictionary, the definition of an herb is "a plant or plant part valued for its medicinal, savory, or aromatic qualities."[5]

Also included in this chapter is information on a few of the other ingredients commonly used in making herbal remedies. The following entries include plant descriptions, botanical names, medicinal properties, precautions and contraindications, and other details.

Angelica

Angelica has been prized for centuries as a versatile culinary herb. Used for everything from soups and stews to candied

5. *Webster's Third New International Dictionary of the English Language* (1981), 1058.

decorations for cakes, it also flavors alcoholic drinks such as Benedictine. Angelica is used medicinally for a range of ailments.

Angelica is a statuesque plant that reaches five to eight feet tall. It has broad leaves and tiny white or greenish flowers that grow in globe-shaped clusters. Ribbed on one side, the seeds are brownish-yellow when ripe. The yellowish-gray root is thick and fleshy.

Botanical names: Angelica archangelica, syn. *A. officinalis*
Also known as: Angelic herb, garden angelica, wild celery, wild parsnip
Parts used: Leaves, seeds, roots
Precautions and contraindications: Avoid during pregnancy and while breastfeeding; avoid with diabetes; use in moderation; roots and seeds may cause sun sensitivity
Medicinal properties: Antibacterial, antifungal, anti-inflammatory, antiseptic, antispasmodic, antiviral, diuretic, expectorant
Used for: Arthritis, bladder infection, bloating, bronchitis, common cold, congestion, cough, cuts and abrasions, edema and lymphedema, fever, flatulence, gout, headache, heartburn/GERD, indigestion, insomnia and sleep, irritable bowel syndrome (IBS), menstrual cramps, nerve pain, nervous tension, psoriasis, sinusitis, stomach pain, stress and anxiety

Black Cohosh

Mostly known for its use in dealing with menopausal and menstrual discomforts, black cohosh can also ease arthritic pain and other ailments. It does not have any culinary use.

Reaching four to six feet tall, black cohosh puts on a show from mid to late summer with white star-shaped flowers that bloom on branching stalks. It has dark green compound leaves and knotty roots that range from dark brown to black.

Botanical names: Actaea racemosa, syn. *Cimicifuga racemosa*
Also known as: Black snakeroot, bugbane, squawroot
Parts used: Roots
Precautions and contraindications: Avoid during pregnancy and while breastfeeding; may cause stomach upset or headache; use for six months or less; check with your doctor before using if you are on prescription medications; should not be given to children under the age of eighteen. Black cohosh is not related to and should not be confused with blue cohosh (*Caulophyllum thalictroides*)
Medicinal properties: Anti-inflammatory, antispasmodic, astringent, diuretic, estrogenic, expectorant, sedative
Used for: Acne, arthritis, asthma, bronchitis, cough, headache, hot flashes and night sweats, insect bites and beestings, headache, low back pain, menopausal discomforts, menstrual cramps, migraine, muscle spasm and cramp, premenstrual syndrome (PMS), rheumatoid arthritis, shin splints, sore throat

Burdock

Rich in vitamins and minerals, all parts of the burdock plant are edible and commonly used as vegetables in Asia. Cooling and detoxifying, burdock has been used in Western, Ayurvedic, and traditional Chinese medicine for centuries.

A biennial plant, burdock consists of a rosette of basal leaves in its first year. In its second year, stems with dull green, heart-shaped leaves shoot up to six feet tall. Clusters of thistle-like pink or purple flowers grow atop the spiny globes of burs.

Botanical name: Arctium lappa
Also known as: Beggar's buttons, burweed, greater burdock
Parts used: Roots, leaves
Precautions and contraindications: Avoid during pregnancy and while breastfeeding; avoid if sensitive to plants in the Asteraceae/Compositae (aster/daisy) family; avoid when on medications that slow blood clotting; do not give to children under the age of eighteen
Medicinal properties: Antibacterial, antifungal, anti-inflammatory, antiseptic, antiviral, diuretic
Used for: Acne, arthritis, bladder infection, boils and carbuncles, bruises, common cold, constipation, dandruff, eczema, edema and lymphedema, flatulence, gout, poison ivy/oak/sumac, prostatitis, psoriasis, ringworm, sciatica, sore throat, sties and chalazia, tonsillitis

Dandelion

The bane of those who want a perfect lawn, the dandelion has both culinary and medicinal uses. It is used as a flavor component in a wide range of commercial products such as beverages, cheeses, and baked goods. The roots and leaves are high in minerals and vitamins, aid digestion, and support kidney health.

Jagged, lance-shaped leaves form a rosette base from which leafless stems rise. The golden flower discs turn to puffy, round seed heads. Individual seeds are dispersed on the wind like little parachutes. The long taproot resembles a skinny carrot.

Botanical name: Taraxacum officinale
Also known as: Bitterwort, blowball, lion's-tooth, wild endive
Parts used: Roots, leaves
Precautions and contraindications: Avoid during pregnancy and while breastfeeding; do not use with gallbladder problems; the white latex fluid contained in the whole plant may cause a reaction for those with allergies to plants in the Asteraceae/Compositae (aster/daisy) family; avoid during antibiotic treatment
Medicinal properties: Antibacterial, anti-inflammatory, antimicrobial, diuretic
Used for: Acne, arthritis, bladder infection, bloating, boils and carbuncles, constipation, eczema, edema and lymphedema, goiter, gout, hangover, hemorrhoids, indigestion, mastitis, premenstrual syndrome (PMS), psoriasis, rheumatoid arthritis, shin splints

Feverfew

As its name suggests, this herb has been traditionally used for treating fever. Nowadays, it is best known for dealing with migraines, especially as a preventative when taken at the first hint that one is starting. Feverfew has very few culinary uses because of its bitter taste.

Sometimes used as an ornamental plant, feverfew is a perennial that grows between one and two feet tall. Its white daisy-like flowers with yellow centers bloom from early to midsummer and into the autumn. The deeply lobed leaflets range from dark to yellowish-green.

Botanical names: Tanacetum parthenium, syn. *Chrysanthemum parthenium, Matricaria parthenium*

Also known as: Bachelor's buttons, false chamomile, wild chamomile

Parts used: Leaves

Precautions and contraindications: Avoid during pregnancy and while breastfeeding; avoid when taking blood-thinning medications and with bleeding disorders; avoid if sensitive to plants in the Asteraceae/Compositae (aster/daisy) family

Medicinal properties: Analgesic, antihistamine, anti-inflammatory, antispasmodic, nervine

Used for: Arthritis, earache, fever, headache, low back pain, menstrual cramps, mental fatigue, migraine, muscle soreness and stiffness, nervous tension, rheumatoid arthritis, shin splints

Hyssop

Hyssop is a powerful herb with antiviral and antibacterial properties, making it effective for a range of respiratory ailments. Like many herbs in the mint family, hyssop comes to the rescue for digestive issues. It has some culinary use as a seasoning in stews, stuffing, and gravies.

With upright angular stems, hyssop grows to about two feet tall. The leaves are dark green and lance-shaped. Tiny purple-blue flowers grow in whorls at the ends of the stems and bloom from midsummer to early autumn.

Botanical name: Hyssopus officinalis
Also known as: Hedge hyssop
Parts used: Leaves, stems, flowers
Precautions and contraindications: Avoid during pregnancy and while breastfeeding; avoid in children under the age of eighteen; use in small doses for short periods of time
Medicinal properties: Antibacterial, anti-inflammatory, antiseptic, antispasmodic, antiviral, astringent, diuretic, expectorant
Used for: Acne, asthma, bloating, bronchitis, bruises, burns and scalds, catarrh, common cold, congestion, cough, cuts and abrasions, fever, flatulence, flu, indigestion, laryngitis, menstrual cramps, muscle soreness and stiffness, nervous tension, sinusitis, sore throat, stomach pain, stress and anxiety, tonsillitis

Lavender

While this beloved garden plant is most widely known for calming and soothing nerves, these properties also extend to the digestive system. It is used sparingly to flavor salads, desserts, jelly, jam, honey, and other dishes.

Lavender is a bushy evergreen shrub that reaches two to three feet tall and wide. Blooming from midsummer to early autumn, its small purplish flowers grow in whorls atop leafless spikes. The slightly fuzzy leaves are narrow and gray-green or silvery-green.

Botanical names: Lavandula angustifolia, syn. *L. officinalis*
Also known as: Common lavender, English lavender, true lavender
Parts used: Leaves, flowers
Precautions and contraindications: Do not use when taking sedative medications
Medicinal properties: Analgesic, antibacterial, antifungal, anti-inflammatory, antimicrobial, antiseptic, antispasmodic, antiviral, diuretic, nervine, sedative
Used for: Acne, athlete's foot, bloating, boils and carbuncles, bruises, burns and scalds, cold sores, common cold, cuts and abrasions, dermatitis, earache, eczema, flatulence, flu, head lice, headache, hemorrhoids, hives, indigestion, insect bites and beestings, insomnia and sleep, jock itch, laryngitis, menopausal discomforts, menstrual cramps, migraine, muscle soreness and stiffness, nervous tension, psoriasis, ringworm, scabies, sciatica, sinusitis, sore throat, sprains and strains, stress and anxiety, sunburn, temporomandibular joint (TMJ) pain, tonsillitis, vaginitis

Lemongrass

The leaves and stems of this plant are used to add a lemony flavor to stews, stir-fries, salsa, and other dishes. Medicinally, it supports the digestive system and is an effective treatment for a range of ailments. Lemongrass not only soothes insect bites, but when used in advance of an outing, it helps repel bugs, too.

Lemongrass grows in large, dense clumps that can reach up to five feet tall and four feet wide. It has long narrow leaf blades and tiny green flowers that grow atop branching stalks. The plant has a lemony fragrance.

Botanical name: Cymbopogon citratus, syn. *Andropogon citratus*
Also known as: Citronella grass, West Indian lemongrass
Parts used: Leaves
Precautions and contraindications: Avoid during pregnancy and while breastfeeding
Medicinal properties: Analgesic, antibacterial, antifungal, anti-inflammatory, antispasmodic, diuretic, expectorant
Used for: Acne, arthritis, athlete's foot, bursitis and tendonitis, cough, fever, flatulence, gingivitis, head lice, headache, indigestion, insect bites and beestings, jock itch, mental fatigue, muscle soreness and stiffness, nervous tension, ringworm, scabies, shin splints, sore throat, sprains and strains, stomach pain, stress and anxiety, vaginitis

Mullein

While mullein (rhymes with sullen) is widely known for treating respiratory ailments, it is also effective in strengthening the nervous and urinary systems, relieving pain, and fighting infection. It does not have any culinary use.

Mullein is a biennial plant with a large rosette of velvety, blue-green leaves. Reaching almost ten feet tall, the spire of flowers develops in the second year. From June to September, its yellow flowers bloom a few at a time.

Botanical name: Verbascum thapsus

Also known as: Flannelleaf, great mullein, velvet plant

Parts used: Leaves, flowers, roots

Precautions and contraindications: Avoid during pregnancy and while breastfeeding

Medicinal properties: Antibacterial, anti-inflammatory, antiseptic, antispasmodic, antiviral, diuretic, expectorant

Used for: Arthritis, asthma, bladder infection, boils and carbuncles, bronchitis, bruises, bursitis and tendonitis, canker sores, catarrh, common cold, congestion, cough, cuts and abrasions, diarrhea, earache, flu, gingivitis, gout, hemorrhoids, indigestion, insect bites and beestings, insomnia and sleep, kidney stones, laryngitis, low back pain, muscle soreness and stiffness, nervous tension, sore throat, swollen glands/lymph nodes, tonsillitis

Nettle

Often regarded as just a weed, nettle is high in vitamins, iron, minerals, and other nutrients. The leaves can be used as a substitute for spinach; cooking renders the plant's sting harmless. Nettle promotes general well-being and is a tonic for the male and female reproductive systems.

Nettle reaches about six feet tall and has heavily veined, toothed leaves. Small whorls of white or green flowers grow at the stem tips and the leaf axils. The stems and leaves are covered with bristly hairs that inject an irritant when brushed against. The irritant causes a burning, itching sensation that can last up to twelve hours.

Botanical name: Urtica dioica
Also known as: Common nettle, stinging nettle
Parts used: Leaves, roots
Precautions and contraindications: May interact with high blood pressure, sedative, and diabetes medications
Medicinal properties: Antiallergenic, antihistamine, anti-inflammatory, astringent, diuretic, styptic
Used for: Arthritis, asthma, bladder infection, bursitis and tendonitis, cuts and abrasions, dermatitis, eczema, fever, goiter, gout, hay fever, hemorrhoids, hives, insect bites and beestings, kidney stones, menopausal discomforts, mental fatigue, muscle soreness and stiffness, premenstrual syndrome (PMS), prostatitis, rheumatoid arthritis, sprain and strain

St. John's Wort

Calming and restorative for the nervous system, this herb's antiviral and astringent properties provide relief for a wide range of ailments. The antibacterial properties of St. John's wort aid in fighting infection. It has had limited culinary use as flavoring for beverages.

St. John's wort is a shrubby plant that reaches two to three feet tall. It has pale green leaves and bright yellow, star-shaped flowers that grow in clusters at the ends of branches. The flowers bloom from mid to late summer and have a light lemon-like scent.

Botanical name: Hypericum perforatum
Also known as: Goatweed, rosin rose, sweet amber
Parts used: Leaves, flowers, buds

Precautions and contraindications: Do not take internally during pregnancy and while breastfeeding; when taking prescription medications, consult your doctor before using

Medicinal properties: Antibacterial, antihistamine, anti-inflammatory, antispasmodic, antiviral, astringent, expectorant, nervine

Used for: Arthritis, bladder infection, bruises, burns and scalds, carpal tunnel syndrome, catarrh, cold sores, congestion, cuts and abrasions, dermatitis, eczema, hay fever, headache, hemorrhoids, insect bites and beestings, insomnia and sleep, laryngitis, mastitis, menopausal discomforts, menstrual cramps, muscle soreness and stiffness, nerve pain, nervous tension, postpartum blues, premenstrual syndrome (PMS), psoriasis, sciatica, seasonal affective disorder (SAD), shingles, sinusitis, sprains and strains, stress and anxiety, sunburn, temporomandibular joint (TMJ) pain, varicose veins

Valerian

Most widely known as a sleep aid and boon for dealing with insomnia, valerian eases stress and anxiety and provides support for the nervous system. Its antispasmodic properties relieve menstrual cramps and nervous indigestion. While its odor is disagreeable, those who brave its bitter taste swear by its effectiveness.

Reaching three to five feet tall, valerian has dark green leaves and small white flowers that grow in dense clusters. The pale brown root is an upright rhizome with fibrous roots extending outward.

Botanical name: Valeriana officinalis

Also known as: Common valerian, garden heliotrope

Parts used: Roots

Precautions and contraindications: Avoid during pregnancy and while breastfeeding; avoid if you have liver problems; use in moderation; large doses can cause dizziness, headache, stupor, and vomiting; avoid using for prolonged periods (use for two or three weeks at a time, then take a break for at least one week); for some, it may stimulate rather than relax

Medicinal properties: analgesic, anti-inflammatory, antispasmodic, sedative

Used for: Arthritis, headache, indigestion, insomnia and sleep, low back pain, menopausal discomforts, menstrual cramps, mental fatigue, migraine, muscle soreness and stiffness, muscle spasm and cramp, nerve pain, nervous tension, rheumatoid arthritis, sciatica, sprains and strains, stomach pain, stress and anxiety, temporomandibular joint (TMJ) pain

Yarrow

While yarrow's fame is related to its styptic properties and for healing wounds, it is effective for a wider repertoire of ailments. Like spearmint, it is an amphoteric herb that does what is needed. It can stimulate or sedate; it can help bring on menses or curb heavy bleeding.

Yarrow is a slender plant with branching stems that grows one to three feet tall. Its fern-like leaves are covered with soft hairs. Blooming from midsummer to autumn, its small white to pinkish flowers grow in wide umbel clusters.

Botanical name: Achillea millefolium
Also known as: Bloodwort, common yarrow, thousand-leaf
Parts used: Leaves, flowers
Precautions and contraindications: Avoid during pregnancy and while breastfeeding; may cause allergic reaction in those sensitive to plants in the Asteraceae/Compositae (aster/daisy) family; large doses may induce headache; use in moderation; do not use when taking medications that slow blood clotting; may increase skin sensitivity to sunlight
Medicinal properties: Antibacterial, anti-inflammatory, antiseptic, antispasmodic, antiviral, astringent, diuretic, styptic
Used for: Acne, bladder infection, boils and carbuncles, bruises, common cold, cuts and abrasions, eczema, fever, flu, hemorrhoids, indigestion, laryngitis, menstrual cramps, muscle soreness and stiffness, rheumatoid arthritis, sore throat, sprains and strains, stomach pain, varicose veins

Other Common Remedy Ingredients

Being familiar with the other major ingredients included in recipes will help you make the best selection for your preparations. In addition to serving as a base for herbal remedies, the following ingredients have some healing properties of their own. Also included in this section is information on what to look for when purchasing some of these ingredients.

Aloe Vera

Aloe vera is a familiar houseplant that is often kept in the kitchen for the first aid treatment of burns. It is a perennial plant with succulent leaves that can grow up to two feet long from a center base. The leaves contain a pale, translucent gel that has a faint herby scent. A yellow juice called *bitter aloe* is exuded at the base of the leaves when they are cut. Bitter aloe is also found just under the skin of the leaves. Unlike the gel, it can be unpleasantly smelly and should not be used on the skin or ingested.

When purchasing aloe gel, look for organic products. Check for the terms *inner leaf* and *whole leaf*. Inner leaf indicates that only the aloe gel was used; whole leaf may contain some bitter aloe. Also, check the ingredients for parabens, fragrance oils (which are not essential oils), and petrochemicals. Aloe gel has an approximate shelf life of six months.

Botanical names: Aloe vera, syn. *A. barbadensis, A. vulgaris*
Parts used: Gel
Precautions and contraindications: Topical use of the gel is generally regarded as safe
Medicinal properties: Anesthetic, antibacterial, anti-inflammatory, antimicrobial, antiseptic, astringent
Used for: Acne, arthritis, burns and scalds, bursitis and tendonitis, chilblains, cuts and abrasions, dandruff, dermatitis, eczema, hemorrhoids, hives, insect bites and beestings, mastitis, menopausal discomforts, poison ivy/oak/sumac, psoriasis, rheumatoid arthritis, scabies, shingles, sunburn, warts

Beeswax

Beeswax is a substance secreted by bees that they use to form the structure of honeycombs. When used medicinally, beeswax protects the skin while allowing it to breathe. Containing vitamins A and E, it aids cell regeneration and nourishes the skin.

When purchasing beeswax, make sure it is filtered and cosmetic or organic grade. Unfiltered wax contains some pollen, honey, and debris from the hive. In addition to removing these substances, filtering conditions the wax so it mixes more easily and evenly with oils.

Botanical name: Cera alba
Precautions and contraindications: Topical use is generally regarded as safe
Medicinal properties: Antiallergenic, antibacterial, anti-inflammatory, antimicrobial, antiseptic
Used for: Acne, boils and carbuncles, bruises, burns and scalds, cuts and abrasions, dermatitis, eczema, hemorrhoids, insect bites and beestings, psoriasis, sunburn

Cocoa Butter

As expected, cocoa butter comes from the cacao tree, a small tropical evergreen. Butter is made from the seeds that are encased within large, reddish-yellow seedpods. The seeds are also referred to as beans. Unrefined cocoa butter is yellowish and has a faint chocolatey scent. Cocoa butter has a shelf life of two to three years.

When purchasing cocoa butter, read the label to make sure you are getting just the butter. Some products labeled as cocoa butter may contain paraffin, petroleum, lanolin, fragrance oils (which are not essential oils), and artificial dyes.

Botanical name: Theobroma cacao
Parts used: Seeds

Precautions and contraindications: Topical use is generally regarded as safe
Medicinal properties: Anti-inflammatory
Used for: Burns and scalds, dermatitis, eczema, psoriasis, sunburn

Oils

Soothing for the skin, herb-infused oils can be used medicinally for massage and bath oils and for making salves and ointments. They also have some healing properties of their own. Following is information on three popular oils.

Coconut Oil

The coconut palm tree has been used for culinary and medicinal purposes worldwide for thousands of years. It still plays a role in traditional medicines, such as Chinese and Ayurveda, and is the subject of ongoing scientific research.

There are two types of coconut oil on the market: refined, also known as Fractionated Coconut Oil (FCO); and unrefined, also known as Virgin Coconut Oil (VCO). The refined oil is odorless and colorless and has reduced healing properties. Unrefined coconut oil is pale yellow or whitish-yellow, has a distinctive coconut aroma, and is a solid at temperatures below 70°F (21°C). It is rich in essential fatty acids, minerals, and vitamins. Coconut oil is highly stable and has an indefinite shelf life.

Botanical name: Cocos nucifera
Parts used: The white lining inside the nut, known as coconut meat

Precautions and contraindications: Topical use is generally regarded as safe

Medicinal properties: Antibacterial, antifungal, anti-inflammatory, antimicrobial, antiviral

Used for: Acne, athlete's foot, cold sores, dandruff, dermatitis, eczema, head lice, hemorrhoids, hives, insect bites and beestings, jock itch, psoriasis, ringworm, sunburn

Jojoba Oil

Found at higher elevations, jojoba is a desert shrub that can live more than a hundred years. Its fruit capsules contain one to three seeds, which are also known as nuts and beans.

Technically, jojoba is a liquid wax. It has a clear golden color, a softly nutty and slightly sweet aroma, and a light texture. It is a liquid at room temperature but solidifies at 50°F (10°C). It is particularly good for the skin because of its similarity to the body's natural oil, sebum. Jojoba oil is highly stable and has an indefinite shelf life.

Botanical name: Simmondsia chinensis

Also known as: Coffeebush, deer nut, wild hazel

Parts used: Seeds

Precautions and contraindications: Topical use is generally regarded as safe

Medicinal properties: Antibacterial, antifungal, anti-inflammatory, antimicrobial, antiseptic, antiviral

Used for: Acne, athlete's foot, cold sores, cuts and abrasions, dandruff, eczema, insect bites and beestings, psoriasis, sunburn, warts

Olive Oil

Produced from a small, gnarly evergreen tree, olive has been one of the most important oils since ancient times for medicinal, culinary, and lighting purposes. Rich in minerals, vitamins, proteins, and essential fatty acids, it is regarded as one of the healthiest oils for the diet. Topically, it helps nourish and protect the skin.

To get the most for healing, buy extra-virgin, cold-pressed oil. The term *virgin* means that the oil came from the first pressing and *extra virgin* means that it is the highest grade. Olive oil has a dark greenish color and an oily texture. It has a shelf life of up to two years.

Botanical name: Olea europaea
Also known as: Common olive
Parts used: Fruit
Precautions and contraindications: Generally regarded as safe
Medicinal properties: Antibacterial, anti-inflammatory
Used for: Bruises, burns and scalds, cuts and abrasions, dandruff, insect bites and beestings, sunburn

Witch Hazel

The witch hazel product commonly available in pharmacies and supermarkets in the United States is a distillate that is produced by steam distillation of the twigs and branches. Although it is milder than a witch hazel extract, it retains the plant's astringent properties.[6] Witch hazel usually contains 14 to 15 percent alcohol, which acts as a preservative. It has a shelf life of two to three years.

The hallmark of this shrubby tree is its yellow flowers that bloom in late autumn. Resembling crinkled ribbons, these spidery flowers on bare branches brighten dull autumn and winter landscapes.

Botanical name: Hamamelis virginiana

Also known as: American witch hazel, spotted alder, winterbloom

Parts used: Twigs, branches

Precautions and contraindications: Topical use is generally regarded as safe

Medicinal properties: Anti-inflammatory, antiseptic, astringent

Used for: Acne, bruises, cuts and abrasions, eczema, hemorrhoids, hives, insect bites and beestings, poison ivy/oak/sumac, psoriasis, sprains and strains, varicose veins

---

6. Witch hazel extract is created through the extraction process, which involves treating plant material with a solvent (usually alcohol). It is made from the leaves and bark, which are high in tannins that give it a highly astringent and drying effect. Extracts are often distilled once or twice to remove some of the tannins.

conclusion

Far from being an outdated form of medicine, the use of herbal remedies and other traditional methods have withstood the test of time. Herbal remedies help us avoid putting more chemicals into and onto our bodies than we have to. They also help us avoid the range of binders, fillers, and preservatives in many over-the-counter remedies that can cause negative side effects.

Herbs offer a holistic way of dealing with common basic health issues because they work with the body to heal and strengthen, establish wellness, and support ongoing good health. As mentioned, we must keep safety in mind. While herbs are natural substances, they are powerful and must be used properly. We must also be aware of their limits and work with our doctors to create a blend of traditional and conventional medicine that works best for ourselves and our families.

When beginning your journey with herbal remedies, it takes more work than simply grabbing a product at the store. Not only is it important to keep track of the ingredients and the amounts used while preparing remedies, it is also important to chart the effectiveness of the dosages we take. This is especially true when working with an herb for the first time. However, over time it will be an easy matter to refer to your notes. While using herbal remedies takes a little more effort, the experience is rewarding in that it supports our ability to be proactive and to take charge of our health.

appendix a

Herbs for Ailments, Conditions, and Support for Good Health

This appendix provides a quick reference guide for which herbs and other ingredients to use for various ailments and conditions. In addition, it will help you get the most from the herbs you have on hand. When using the recipes provided in this book, you can refer to this section to find substitutes for herbs that you may not have. Of course, remedies can be made with only one herb, too.

Acne

Herbs: Black cohosh, burdock, chamomile, coriander, dandelion, hyssop, lavender, lemon balm, lemongrass, peppermint, rosemary, sage, spearmint, thyme, yarrow

Other ingredients: Aloe vera, beeswax, coconut oil, jojoba oil, witch hazel

Anxiety: *See* Stress and Anxiety

Arthritis

Herbs: Angelica, bay laurel, black cohosh, burdock, cayenne, chamomile, coriander, dandelion, dill, feverfew, ginger, lemongrass, mullein, nettle, parsley, rosemary, sage, St. John's wort, thyme, turmeric, valerian

Other ingredients: Aloe vera

Asthma

Herbs: Anise, bay laurel, black cohosh, chamomile, dill, fennel, ginger, hyssop, lemon balm, mullein, nettle, oregano, parsley, peppermint, rosemary, sage, spearmint, thyme, turmeric

Athlete's Foot

Herbs: Bay laurel, garlic, lavender, lemongrass, thyme

Other ingredients: Coconut oil, jojoba oil

Beestings: *See* Insect Bites and Beestings

Belching

Herbs: Caraway, chamomile, fennel, ginger, peppermint, spearmint

Bladder Infection

Herbs: Angelica, burdock, dandelion, garlic, ginger, mullein, nettle, parsley, St. John's wort, yarrow

Bloating

Herbs: Angelica, anise, bay laurel, caraway, chamomile, coriander, dandelion, fennel, ginger, hyssop, lavender, peppermint, rosemary, thyme

Boils and Carbuncles

Herbs: Burdock, dandelion, lavender, mullein, sage, thyme, yarrow

Other ingredients: Beeswax

Breastfeeding

Herbs: Anise, caraway, dill, fennel, parsley, sage

Bronchitis

Herbs: Angelica, anise, basil, black cohosh, caraway, coriander, dill, fennel, garlic, hyssop, lemon balm, mullein, oregano, peppermint, rosemary, spearmint, thyme

Bruises

Herbs: Bay laurel, burdock, caraway, fennel, hyssop, lavender, mullein, parsley, rosemary, St. John's wort, thyme, yarrow

Other ingredients: Beeswax, olive oil, witch hazel

Burns and Scalds

Herbs: Chamomile, hyssop, lavender, peppermint, spearmint, St. John's wort

Other ingredients: Aloe vera, beeswax, cocoa butter, olive oil

Bursitis and Tendonitis

Herbs: Cayenne, ginger, lemongrass, mullein, nettle, peppermint, rosemary, turmeric

Other ingredients: Aloe vera

Canker Sores

Herbs: Basil, chamomile, coriander, mullein, rosemary, sage, thyme

Carpal Tunnel Syndrome

Herbs: Bay laurel, cayenne, chamomile, sage, St. John's wort, turmeric

Catarrh

Herbs: Garlic, hyssop, mullein, oregano, sage, St. John's wort, thyme

Chalazia: *See* Sties and Chalazia

Chilblains

Herbs: Cayenne, ginger, spearmint

Other ingredients: Aloe vera

Cold Sores

Herbs: Ginger, lavender, lemon balm, St. John's wort

Other ingredients: Coconut oil, jojoba oil

Colic

Herbs: Caraway, chamomile, dill, fennel, spearmint

Common Cold

Herbs: Angelica, anise, basil, bay laurel, burdock, cayenne, chamomile, dill, garlic, ginger, hyssop, lavender, lemon balm, mullein, oregano, peppermint, rosemary, sage, spearmint, thyme, yarrow

Congestion

Herbs: Angelica, anise, bay laurel, caraway, cayenne, dill, fennel, garlic, ginger, hyssop, lemon balm, mullein, oregano, peppermint, rosemary, sage, spearmint, St. John's wort, thyme

Constipation

Herbs: Basil, burdock, dandelion, dill, ginger, oregano, parsley

Cough

Herbs: Angelica, anise, basil, black cohosh, caraway, coriander, dill, fennel, garlic, ginger, hyssop, lemon balm, lemongrass, mullein, oregano, parsley, peppermint, spearmint, thyme

Cuts and Abrasions

Herbs: Angelica, cayenne, chamomile, garlic, ginger, hyssop, lavender, mullein, nettle, oregano, rosemary, sage, St. John's wort, thyme, turmeric, yarrow

Other ingredients: Aloe vera, beeswax, jojoba oil, olive oil, witch hazel

Dandruff

Herbs: Bay laurel, burdock, chamomile, parsley, rosemary, sage

Other ingredients: Aloe vera, coconut oil, jojoba oil, olive oil

Dermatitis

Herbs: Chamomile, lavender, lemon balm, nettle, St. John's wort

Other ingredients: Aloe vera, beeswax, cocoa butter, coconut oil

Diarrhea

Herbs: Cayenne, coriander, mullein, peppermint, sage, thyme

Earache

Herbs: Chamomile, feverfew, garlic, lavender, mullein, thyme

Eczema

Herbs: Burdock, chamomile, dandelion, lavender, lemon balm, nettle, peppermint, rosemary, St. John's wort, turmeric, yarrow

Other ingredients: Aloe vera, beeswax, cocoa butter, coconut oil, jojoba oil, witch hazel

Edema and Lymphedema

Herbs: Angelica, burdock, coriander, dandelion, fennel, ginger

Eyes, Puffy

Herbs: Chamomile, fennel, parsley, rosemary

Fever

Herbs: Angelica, anise, chamomile, coriander, fennel, feverfew, ginger, hyssop, lemon balm, lemongrass, nettle, peppermint, sage, spearmint, yarrow

Flatulence

Herbs: Angelica, anise, basil, bay laurel, burdock, caraway, cayenne, chamomile, coriander, dill, fennel, ginger, hyssop, lavender, lemon balm, lemongrass, oregano, parsley, peppermint, rosemary, spearmint, thyme, turmeric

Flu

Herbs: Anise, basil, bay laurel, cayenne, garlic, ginger, hyssop, lavender, lemon balm, mullein, oregano, peppermint, rosemary, sage, thyme, yarrow

Gingivitis

Herbs: Basil, lemongrass, mullein, peppermint, sage, spearmint, thyme, turmeric

Goiter

Herbs: Dandelion, garlic, lemon balm, nettle, parsley

Gout

Herbs: Angelica, burdock, cayenne, dandelion, ginger, mullein, nettle, parsley, turmeric

Halitosis

Herbs: Anise, basil, caraway, coriander, dill, parsley, peppermint, rosemary, sage, spearmint, thyme, turmeric

Hangover

Herbs: Cayenne, dandelion, thyme

Hay Fever

Herbs: Chamomile, ginger, nettle, parsley, St. John's wort, thyme

Head Lice

Herbs: Anise, lavender, lemongrass, parsley, thyme
Other ingredients: Coconut oil

Headache

Herbs: Angelica, basil, black cohosh, cayenne, chamomile, coriander, dill, feverfew, ginger, lavender, lemon balm, lemongrass, oregano, parsley, peppermint, rosemary, sage, St. John's wort, thyme, turmeric, valerian

Heartburn/GERD

Herbs: Angelica, caraway, chamomile, coriander, dill, fennel, ginger, lemon balm, peppermint, spearmint

Hemorrhoids

Herbs: Chamomile, coriander, dandelion, dill, lavender, mullein, nettle, sage, St. John's wort, yarrow

Other ingredients: Aloe vera, beeswax, coconut oil, witch hazel

Hives

Herbs: Chamomile, lavender, nettle, parsley, rosemary

Other ingredients: Aloe vera, coconut oil, witch hazel

Hot Flashes and Night Sweats

Herbs: Anise, black cohosh, fennel, sage, spearmint

Indigestion

Herbs: Angelica, anise, basil, bay laurel, caraway, chamomile, coriander, dandelion, dill, fennel, ginger, hyssop, lavender, lemon balm, lemongrass, mullein, oregano, peppermint, rosemary, spearmint, thyme, turmeric, valerian, yarrow

Insect Bites and Beestings

Herbs: Basil, bay laurel, black cohosh, chamomile, fennel, lavender, lemon balm, lemongrass, mullein, nettle, parsley, peppermint, sage, spearmint, St. John's wort

Other ingredients: Aloe vera, beeswax, coconut oil, jojoba oil, olive oil, witch hazel

Insomnia and Sleep

Herbs: Angelica, anise, basil, chamomile, coriander, dill, lavender, lemon balm, mullein, oregano, peppermint, sage, spearmint, St. John's wort, valerian

Irritable Bowel Syndrome (IBS)

Herbs: Angelica, caraway, chamomile, fennel, garlic, lemon balm, peppermint, rosemary

Jock Itch

Herbs: Bay laurel, chamomile, garlic, lavender, lemongrass, thyme

Other ingredients: Coconut oil

Kidney Stones

Herbs: Basil, fennel, mullein, nettle, parsley

Laryngitis

Herbs: Chamomile, fennel, hyssop, lavender, mullein, peppermint, sage, spearmint, St. John's wort, thyme, yarrow

Leukorrhea

Herbs: Basil, sage, turmeric, yarrow

Other ingredients: Aloe vera

Low Back Pain

Herbs: Black cohosh, cayenne, feverfew, ginger, mullein, rosemary, spearmint, thyme, turmeric, valerian

Lymphedema: *See* Edema and Lymphedema

Mastitis

Herbs: Chamomile, dandelion, ginger, parsley, St. John's wort

Other ingredients: Aloe vera

Menopausal Discomforts

Herbs: Anise, black cohosh, chamomile, fennel, lavender, lemon balm, nettle, sage, St. John's wort, thyme, valerian

Other ingredients: Aloe vera

Menstrual Cramps

Herbs: Angelica, anise, black cohosh, caraway, chamomile, coriander, dill, fennel, feverfew, ginger, hyssop, lavender, lemon balm, oregano, parsley, peppermint, rosemary, St. John's wort, thyme, valerian, yarrow

Mental Fatigue

Herbs: Basil, coriander, feverfew, ginger, lemongrass, nettle, peppermint, rosemary, sage, valerian

Migraine

Herbs: Black cohosh, cayenne, feverfew, lavender, lemon balm, oregano, peppermint, rosemary, thyme, valerian

Motion Sickness

Herbs: Basil, cayenne, chamomile, fennel, ginger, oregano, peppermint, spearmint, turmeric

Muscle Soreness and Stiffness

Herbs: Bay laurel, cayenne, chamomile, coriander, feverfew, ginger, hyssop, lavender, lemongrass, mullein, nettle, oregano, peppermint, rosemary, sage, spearmint, St. John's wort, thyme, valerian, yarrow

Muscle Spasm and Cramp

Herbs: Black cohosh, cayenne, chamomile, coriander, peppermint, rosemary, thyme, valerian

Nausea

Herbs: Anise, basil, chamomile, coriander, fennel, ginger, peppermint, spearmint, turmeric

Nerve Pain

Herbs: Angelica, cayenne, chamomile, coriander, ginger, lemon balm, peppermint, St. John's wort, turmeric, valerian

Nervous Tension

Herbs: Angelica, basil, chamomile, coriander, dill, feverfew, hyssop, lavender, lemon balm, lemongrass, mullein, oregano, peppermint, rosemary, sage, St. John's wort, valerian

Night Sweats: *See* Hot Flashes and Night Sweats

Poison Ivy, Poison Oak, and Poison Sumac

Herbs: Burdock

Other ingredients: Aloe vera, witch hazel

Postpartum Blues

Herbs: Anise, caraway, chamomile, dill, fennel, lemon balm, St. John's wort

Premenstrual Syndrome (PMS)

Herbs: Black cohosh, chamomile, dandelion, fennel, ginger, lemon balm, nettle, parsley, St. John's wort, thyme

Prostatitis

Herbs: Burdock, nettle, turmeric

Psoriasis

Herbs: Angelica, burdock, chamomile, dandelion, lavender, lemon balm, St. John's wort, turmeric

Other ingredients: Aloe vera, beeswax, cocoa butter, coconut oil, jojoba oil, witch hazel

Rheumatoid Arthritis

Herbs: Black cohosh, cayenne, chamomile, dandelion, feverfew, ginger, nettle, turmeric, valerian, yarrow

Other ingredients: Aloe vera

Ringworm

Herbs: Burdock, garlic, lavender, lemongrass, thyme, turmeric

Other ingredients: Coconut oil

Scabies

Herbs: Anise, bay laurel, garlic, lavender, lemongrass, thyme
Other ingredients: Aloe vera

Sciatica

Herbs: Bay laurel, burdock, cayenne, chamomile, ginger, lavender, lemon balm, St. John's wort, thyme, valerian

Seasonal Affective Disorder (SAD)

Herbs: Lemon balm, St. John's wort

Shin Splints

Herbs: Anise, black cohosh, cayenne, chamomile, dandelion, feverfew, ginger, lemongrass, thyme

Shingles

Herbs: Cayenne, lemon balm, St. John's wort
Other ingredients: Aloe vera

Sinusitis

Herbs: Angelica, anise, basil, bay laurel, garlic, ginger, hyssop, lavender, lemon balm, peppermint, rosemary, sage, St. John's wort, thyme

Sore Throat

Herbs: Bay laurel, black cohosh, burdock, cayenne, chamomile, fennel, garlic, ginger, hyssop, lavender, lemongrass, mullein, oregano, peppermint, rosemary, sage, spearmint, thyme, yarrow

Sprains and Strains

Herbs: Bay laurel, chamomile, lavender, lemongrass, nettle, oregano, peppermint, rosemary, St. John's wort, thyme, valerian, yarrow

Other ingredients: Witch hazel

Stomach Pain

Herbs: Angelica, anise, basil, caraway, cayenne, chamomile, coriander, dill, fennel, hyssop, lemon balm, lemongrass, peppermint, rosemary, thyme, turmeric, valerian, yarrow

Stress and Anxiety

Herbs: Angelica, anise, basil, chamomile, coriander, ginger, hyssop, lavender, lemon balm, lemongrass, rosemary, spearmint, St. John's wort, valerian

Sties and Chalazia

Herbs: Burdock, chamomile, coriander, thyme, turmeric

Sunburn

Herbs: Chamomile, lavender, peppermint, rosemary, spearmint, St. John's wort

Other ingredients: Aloe vera, beeswax, cocoa butter, coconut oil, jojoba oil, olive oil

Swollen Glands/Lymph Nodes

Herbs: Chamomile, garlic, ginger, mullein, peppermint, rosemary, sage, thyme, turmeric

Temporomandibular Joint (TMJ) Pain

Herbs: Coriander, lavender, oregano, rosemary, St. John's wort, valerian

Tendonitis: *See* Bursitis and Tendonitis

Tonsillitis

Herbs: Burdock, chamomile, garlic, ginger, hyssop, lavender, mullein, oregano, peppermint, sage, thyme

Toothache

Herbs: Chamomile, ginger, peppermint, spearmint, thyme

Vaginitis

Herbs: Bay laurel, garlic, lavender, lemongrass, sage

Varicose Veins

Herbs: Rosemary, St. John's wort, yarrow

Other ingredients: Witch hazel

Warts

Herbs: Basil, garlic, thyme

Other ingredients: Aloe vera, jojoba oil

appendix b

Measurement Equivalents

The following table will help you find the easiest way to measure ingredients for your remedies. A measurement to note is that 16 ounces equals a pound in weight and a pint in volume.

Measurement Equivalents

1 tablespoon = 3 teaspoons
1⁄16 cup = 1 tablespoon
⅛ cup = 2 tablespoons
⅙ cup = 2 tablespoons + 2 teaspoons
¼ cup = 4 tablespoons
⅓ cup = 5 tablespoons + 1 teaspoon
⅜ cup = 6 tablespoons
½ cup = 8 tablespoons
⅔ cup = 10 tablespoons + 2 teaspoons
¾ cup = 12 tablespoons
1 cup = 16 tablespoons or 48 teaspoons

1 ounce = 2 tablespoons

4 ounces = ½ cup

8 ounces = 1 cup

1 pint = 2 cups or 16 ounces

1 quart = 2 pints or 4 cups or 32 ounces

1 gallon = 4 quarts

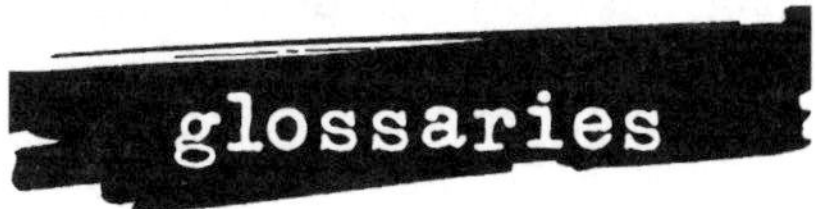

glossaries

Botanical Glossary

Aerial: The parts of a plant that grow aboveground, such as the stems, flowers, and leaves.

Annual: A plant that completes its life cycle in one season.

Basal leaves: The leaves that grow at the base of a plant.

Biennial: A plant with a life cycle of two years.

Compound leaf: A leaf comprised of small leaflets along a common stem.

Cultivar: A variety of plant that is developed and cultivated by humans rather than by natural selection in the wild.

Florets: Tiny individual flowers that grow in a dense cluster and make up a larger flower head.

Flower head: A dense cluster of tiny individual flowers.

Kernel: The inner and softer part of a seed or nut.

Leaf axil: The angle formed by a stem and a smaller leaf stem sprouting from it.

Perennial: A plant with a life cycle of more than two years.

Rhizome: A horizontal underground stem that stores nutrients for a plant. It is often regarded as a type of root.

Spike: A long flower-bearing stem without branches or leaves.

Toothed leaf: A leaf with serrated edges.

Umbel: A common flower head structure with multiple stems radiating from a central stem. Although it can be round like a globe, it most often has the shape of an umbrella.

Whorl: A circular or spiral growth pattern of leaves, needles, or flower petals.

General Glossary

Amphoteric: An herb that can react in different ways according to the situation. It can stimulate or relax, warm or cool.

Balm: A type of preparation with a very firm consistency that forms a protective layer on the skin.

Decoction: A preparation created by simmering the tougher parts of plants in water. These include roots, bark, twigs, seeds, nuts, and dried berries.

Fomentation: A treatment that consists of alternating warm and cool compresses.

Infusion: A preparation created by steeping the aerial parts of a plant in water or oil. Seeds and berries are often included.

Liniment: A preparation for rubbing on the body to soothe pain and stiffness by creating a warming counterirritant.

Maceration: A preparation made by steeping plant material in cold water. It is also called a *cold infusion.*

Ointment: A type of preparation with a slightly firm consistency that forms a protective layer on the skin.

Poultice: A thick herbal paste that is applied topically.

Salve: A type of preparation with a semi-firm consistency that forms a protective layer on the skin.

Sitz bath: A method of bathing in which a person sits in shallow water up to the hips. It is also called a *hip bath.*

Tea: A mild infusion made from the tea plant, *Camellia sinensis.*

Tincture: A preparation usually made with alcohol instead of water or oil.

Tisane: A mild infusion made from any plant except the tea plant (*Camellia sinensis*).

Medical Glossary

Acne: A common skin problem often resulting from bacteria or clogged hair follicles.

Acute: A condition or disease with a rapid onset that lasts for a short period of time.

Analgesic: A substance that relieves pain.

Antiallergenic: A substance that reduces the symptoms of allergies.

Antibacterial: A substance that inhibits the growth of bacteria.

Antifungal: A substance that inhibits the growth of fungus.

Anti-inflammatory: A substance that reduces inflammation.

Antiseptic: A substance that destroys infection-causing bacteria.

Antispasmodic: A substance that relieves muscle spasms and cramping.

Antiviral: A substance that inhibits the growth of a virus.

Arthritis: The inflammation of one or more joints accompanied by pain and stiffness.

Asthma: A chronic lung disease that inflames and narrows the respiratory airways.

Astringent: A substance that dries and contracts organic tissue.

Athlete's foot: A fungal infection on the foot.

Belching: The release of excess air from the stomach through the mouth.

Bloating: A condition caused by excess air in the stomach or intestines that is not passed by belching or flatulence.

Boil: An infection of a hair follicle or oil gland and the surrounding skin.

Bronchitis: The inflammation of the bronchial tubes of the lungs.

Bursitis: The inflammation of the bursae, the fluid sacs that act as cushions in the joints.

Canker sore: A small lesion in the mouth. It is also called an *aphthous ulcer* and *mouth ulcer.*

Carbuncle: A cluster of boils.

Carpal tunnel syndrome: A condition that is characterized by tingling, numbness, and pain in the fingers and hand.

Cartilage: The flexible connective tissue found in many areas of the body. In the joints, it provides cushioning for the bones.

Catarrh: The excessive buildup and discharge of mucus in the nose, sinuses, or throat.

Chalazion: A clogged oil gland on the eyelid.

Chilblains: The painful inflammation of small blood vessels in the skin after exposure to cold.

Chronic: A persistent condition or disease that is long-term.

Cold sores: Blistering sores caused by the herpes simplex virus (HSV). They are also called *fever blisters.*

Colic: A pain in the abdomen caused by intestinal gas or an obstruction.

Congestion: An excess of mucus in the chest or nasal passages due to the common cold, the flu, or allergies.

Constipation: Generally regarded as having three or fewer bowel movements a week.

Dermatitis: Inflammation of the skin that causes it to become reddish, swollen, and itchy or sore.

Diarrhea: Loose, watery, and sometimes frequent bowel movements.

Dyspepsia: The discomfort or pain in the upper abdomen. It is also called *indigestion* and *upset stomach.*

Eczema: The name for a group of skin conditions characterized by a red itchy rash and other symptoms.

Edema: The swelling that occurs when fluid from small blood vessels builds up in the surrounding tissue.

Flatulence: The passing of intestinal gas through the anus.

Fungal infection: A common infection of the skin caused by a fungus. Fungal infections include athlete's foot, jock itch, ringworm, and yeast infections.

Gingivitis: The inflammation, irritation, and redness of the gums around the base of the teeth.

Goiter: The enlargement of the thyroid gland.

Gout: A type of arthritis that occurs when uric acid builds up and causes joint inflammation.

Halitosis: A condition that results from a buildup of bacteria in the mouth. It is commonly known as bad breath.

Hay fever: A seasonal allergy caused by outdoor allergens.

Heartburn/GERD (Gastroeophageal Reflux Disease): A disorder affecting the muscle between the esophagus and stomach.

Hemorrhoids: A condition caused by swollen rectal veins. They are also called *piles.*

Hives: The common name for *urticaria,* which is characterized by swollen pale red patches and welts on the skin.

Irritable Bowel Syndrome (IBS): A disorder that effects the large intestine and impairs the movement of food and waste.

Jock itch: A fungal infection that affects the skin of the genitals, inner thighs, and buttocks.

Laryngitis: The inflammation of the larynx or voice box.

Lumbago: A name used in the past for low back pain.

Lymphedema: The swelling caused by the inability of lymph fluid to flow properly through the lymph vessels and into the bloodstream.

Mastitis: An inflammation of breast tissue that sometimes includes infection.

Motion sickness: A condition most often marked by a queasy stomach and dizziness that can occur with any type of transportation. It is also called *travel sickness* and *seasickness.*

Muscle spasm/cramp: A spasm is the sudden involuntary contraction of a muscle that usually does not last long. A muscle cramp is a sustained spasm.

Nausea: A queasy feeling in the stomach that often precedes vomiting.

Nerve pain: Pain that seems to occur for no obvious reason. It is also called *neuropathic pain.*

Nervine: A substance that restores the nerves and relaxes the nervous system.

Postpartum blues: A condition characterized by mood swings, crying, and sadness following the birth of a baby.

Premenstrual syndrome (PMS): A term that refers to a wide variety of symptoms that occur before and/or during menstruation.

Prostatitis: The inflammation and swelling of the prostate gland.

Psoriasis: A skin condition that causes itchy or sore patches of thick red skin accompanied by silvery scales.

Rheumatism: This term has been used informally for a variety of inflammation and joint pain symptoms. It is no longer used on its own medically to define a disorder or ailment.

Rheumatoid arthritis: A type of inflammatory arthritis in which the immune system mistakenly attacks the joints.

Ringworm: A type of fungal infection that is characterized by a circular rash.

Scabies: A contagious and itchy skin infection caused by the *Sarcoptes scabiei* mite.

Sciatica: Pain or numbness that runs from the lower back down the leg along the pathway of the sciatic nerve.

Seasonal affective disorder (SAD): A type of depression that occurs during the same season each year. It most often occurs in winter.

Shin splints: Pain that occurs along the shin bone at the front of the leg below the knee.

Shingles: An infection caused by the varicella-zoster virus that is characterized by a burning, blistering rash.

Sinusitis: A bacterial or viral infection of the sinuses.

Sprain: A stretch and/or tear of a ligament.

Staph infection: An infection caused by a *Staphylococcus* bacterium.

Stomach pain: A mild to sharp pain or cramp in the stomach or abdomen.

Strain: A stretch and/or tear of a muscle.

Stye: A localized and painful infection on the eyelid. It is known medically as a hordeolum.

Styptic: A substance used externally to stop minor bleeding.

Tendonitis: The irritation or inflammation of a tendon.

Temporomandibular joint (TMJ) pain: Pain that occurs in and/or around the joints of the jaw.

Tonsillitis: The inflammation and infection of the tonsils caused by bacteria or a virus.

Vaginitis: An infection or inflammation of vaginal tissue.

Varicose veins: Enlarged, twisted blood vessels that appear blue and bulging through the skin.

Wart: A benign growth caused by a virus in the top layer of the skin.

bibliography

Arrowsmith, Nancy. *Essential Herbal Wisdom: A Complete Exploration of 50 Remarkable Herbs.* Woodbury, MN: Llewellyn Publications, 2009.

Balch, Phyllis, A. *Prescription for Herbal Healing: An Easy-to-Use A-to-Z Reference to Hundreds of Common Disorders and Their Herbal Remedies*, 2nd ed. New York: Penguin Group, 2012.

Barnes, Joanne, Linda A. Anderson, and J. David Phillipson. *Herbal Medicines*, 3rd ed. London: Pharmaceutical Press-Royal Pharmaceutical Society (RPS) Publishing, 2007.

Barrett, Judy. *What Can I do with My Herbs? How to Grow, Use & Enjoy These Versatile Plants.* College Station, TX: Texas A & M University Press, 2009.

Bedson, Paul. *The Complete Family Guide to Natural Healing.* Dingley, Australia: Hinkler Books Pty. Ltd., 2005.

Bonar, Ann. *Herbs: A Complete Guide to the Cultivation and Use of Wild and Domesticated Herbs.* New York: MacMillan Publishing Co., 1985.

Bone, Kerry. *A Clinical Guide to Blending Liquid Herbs: Herbal Formulations for the Individual Patient*. St. Louis, MO: Churchill Livingston, 2003.

Bonewit-West, Kathy, Sue Hunt, and Edith Applegate. *Today's Medical Assistant: Clinical & Administrative Procedures*, 3rd ed. St. Louis, MO: Elsevier Inc., 2016.

Braun, Lesley, and Marc Cohen. *Herbs and Natural Supplements: An Evidence-based Guide*. 3rd ed. Sydney, Australia: Elsevier, 2010.

Brown, Kathleen, and Jeanine Pollak. *Herbal Teas for Lifelong Health*. North Adams, MA: Storey Publishing, 1999.

Bruton-Seal, Julie, and Mathew Seal. *Backyard Medicine: Harvest and Make Your Own Herbal Remedies*. New York: Skyhorse Publishing, 2009.

Campion, Kitty. *The Family Medical Herbal: A Complete Guide to Maintaining Health and Treating Illness with Plants*. New York: Barnes & Noble Books, 1988.

Castleman, Michael. *The Healing Herbs: The Ultimate Guide to the Curative Power of Nature's Medicines*. New York: Bantam Books, 1995.

_____. *The New Healing Herbs: The Classic Guide to Nature's Best Medicines*. Emmaus, PA: Rodale Press, Inc., 2001.

_____. *The New Healing Herbs: The Essential Guide to More Than 125 of Nature's Most Potent Herbal Remedies*. Emmaus, PA: Rodale Press, Inc., 2009.

Centers for Disease Control and Prevention, "Shingles (Herpes Zoster)." Atlanta, GA: U.S. Department of Health and Human Services, Centers for Disease Control and Prevention. https://www.cdc.gov/shingles/about/index.html#, accessed 1/17/19.

Chevallier, Andrew. *The Encyclopedia of Medicinal Plants: A Practical Reference Guide to Over 550 Key Herbs and Their Medicinal Uses.* New York: Dorling Kindersley Publishing, Inc., 1996.

_____. *Herbal Remedies.* New York: Dorling Kindersley Publishing, Inc., 2007.

Couplan, François. *The Encyclopedia of Edible Plants of North America: Nature's Green Feast.* New Canaan, CT: Keats Publishing, 1998.

Crawford, Amanda McQuade. *Discover Nature's Wonderful Secrets Just for Women.* Roseville, CA: Three Rivers Press, 1997.

Cumo, Christopher, ed., *Encyclopedia of Cultivated Plants: From Acacia to Zinnia*, vol. 3. Santa Barbara, CA: ABC-CLIO, 2013.

Duke, James A. *The Green Pharmacy.* Emmaus, PA: Rodale Press, 1997.

_____. *Duke's Handbook of Medicinal Herbs*, 2nd ed. Boca Raton, FL: CRC Press, LLC, 2002.

_____. *CRC Handbook of Medicinal Spices.* Boca Raton, FL: CRC Press, LLC, 2003.

Editorial Staff. *Webster's Third New International Dictionary of the English Language*, Unabridged, vol. 2. Chicago: Encyclopedia Britannica, Inc., 1981.

Fetrow, Charles W., and Juan R. Avila. *The Complete Guide to Herbal Medicines.* New York: Pocket Books, 2000.

Fife, Bruce. *Coconut Cures: Preventing and Treating Common Health Problems with Coconut.* Colorado Springs, CO: Piccadilly Books, Ltd., 2005.

Foster, Steven, and Rebecca L. Johnson. *National Geographic Desk Reference to Nature's Medicine*. Washington, DC: National Geographic Society, 2008.

Fulder, Stephen, and John Blackwood. *Garlic: Nature's Original Remedy*, rev. ed. Rochester, VT: Healing Arts Press, 2000.

Gladstar, Rosemary. *Medicinal Herbs: A Beginner's Guide*. North Adams, MA: Storey Publishing, 2012.

Goldstein, Myrna Chandler, and Mark A. Goldstein. *Healthy Oils: Fact versus Fiction*. Santa Barbara, CA: Greenwood, 2014.

Green, Aliza. *Field Guide to Herbs & Spices: How to Identify, Select, and Use Virtually Every Seasoning at the Market*. Philadelphia: Quirk Productions, Inc., 2006.

Griggs, Barbara. *The Home Herbal: A Handbook of Simple Remedies*. London: Robert Hale Ltd., 1986.

Groves, Maria Noël. *Body into Balance: An Herbal Guide to Holistic Self-Care*. North Adams, MA: Storey Publishing, 2016.

Hauser, Stephen Crane, ed. *Mayo Clinic on Digestive Health*, 3rd ed. Rochester, MN: Mayo Clinic, 2011.

Hobbs, Christopher, and Kathi Keville. *Women's Herbs, Women's Health*, rev. ed. Summertown, TN: Botanica Press, 2007.

Insel, Paul, Don Ross, Kimberley McMahon, and Melissa Bernstein. *Discovering Nutrition*, 6th ed. Burlington, MA: Jones & Bartlett Learning, 2019.

Kalyn, Wayne, ed. *The Healing Power of Vitamins, Minerals, and Herbs*. Pleasantville, NY: The Reader's Digest Association, Inc., 2000.

Kowalchik, Claire, and William H. Hylton, eds. *Rodale's Illustrated Encyclopedia of Herbs*. Emmaus, PA: Rodale Press, Inc., 1998.

Lad, Vasant. *The Complete Book of Ayurvedic Home Remedies: Based on the Timeless Wisdom of India's 5,000-year-old Medical System*. New York: Three Rivers Press, 1999.

Le Vay, David, G. A. G. Mitchell, and James Scott Robson, "Renal System," *Encyclopaedia Britannica*. Chicago: Encyclopaedia Britannica, Inc., 6/15/18, https://www.britannica.com/science/human-renal-system, accessed 12/12/18.

Lust, John. *The Herb Book: The Most Complete Catalog of Herbs Ever Publishe*d. Mineola, NY: Dover Publications, Inc., 2014.

MacGill, Markus. "Arthritis and Rheumatism: What's the difference?" *Medical News Today*. MediLexicon, International, 7/17/17, https://www.medicalnewstoday.com/articles/7625.php, accessed 12/4/18.

Madison, Deborah. *The Illustrated Encyclopedia of Fruits, Vegetables, and Herbs: History, Botany, Cuisine*. New York: Chartwell Books, 2017.

Mayo Clinic Staff. "Anxiety Disorders." Mayoclinic.org. Rochester, MN: Mayo Clinic School of Medicine. https://www.mayoclinic.org/diseases-conditions/anxiety/symptoms-causes/syc-20350961, accessed 1/9/19.

Mayo Clinic Staff. "Arthritis." Mayoclinic.org. Rochester, MN: Mayo Clinic School of Medicine. https://www.mayoclinic.org/diseases-conditions/arthritis/symptoms-causes/syc-20350772, accessed 11/3/18.

Mayo Clinic Staff. "Kidney Stones." Mayoclinic.org. Rochester, MN: Mayo Clinic School of Medicine. https://www.mayoclinic.org/diseases-conditions/kidney-stones/symptoms-causes/syc-20355755, accessed 11/12/18.

Mayo Clinic Staff. "Poison Ivy Rash." Mayoclinic.org. Rochester, MN: Mayo Clinic School of Medicine. https://www.mayoclinic.org/diseases-conditions/poison-ivy/diagnosis-treatment/drc-20376490, accessed 1/16/19.

Mayo Clinic Staff. "Prostatitis." Mayoclinic.org. Rochester, MN: Mayo Clinic School of Medicine. https://www.mayoclinic.org/diseases-conditions/prostatitis/symptoms-causes/syc-20355766, accessed 12/11/18.

Mayo Clinic Staff, "Seasonal Affective Disorder (SAD)." Mayoclinic.org. Rochester, MN: Mayo Clinic School of Medicine. https://www.mayoclinic.org/diseases-conditions/seasonal-affective-disorder/symptoms-causes/syc-20364651, accessed 1/5/19.

Mayo Clinic Staff. "Sprains and Strains." Mayoclinic.org. Rochester, MN: Mayo Clinic School of Medicine. https://www.mayoclinic.org/diseases-conditions/sprains-and-strains/symptoms-causes/syc-20377938, accessed 12/4/18.

Mayo Clinic Staff. "Stress Management." Mayoclinic.org. Rochester, MN: Mayo Clinic School of Medicine. https://www.mayoclinic.org/healthy-lifestyle/stress-management/basics/stress-basics/hlv-20049495, accessed 1/9/19.

McDowell, Julie, ed. *Encyclopedia of Human Body Systems*. Santa Barbara, CA: Greenwood, 2010.

McBride, Kami. *The Herbal Kitchen: 50 Easy-to-Find Herbs and Over 250 Recipes to Bring Lasting Health to Your Family*. San Francisco: Conari Press, 2010.

McIntyre, Anne. *Herbs for Common Ailments*. New York: Fireside, 1992.

_____. *Herbal Treatment of Children: Western and Ayurvedic Perspectives*. Philadelphia: Elsevier, Ltd., 2005.

McKenna, Dennis J., Kenneth Jones, and Kerry Hughes. *Botanical Medicines: The Desk Reference for Major Herbal Supplements*, 2nd ed. New York: Routledge, 2011.

McVicar, Jekka. *Grow Herbs: An Inspiring Guide to Growing and Using Herbs*. London: Dorling Kindersley Ltd., 2010.

Murray, Michael, Joseph Pizzorno, and Lara Pizzorno. *The Encyclopedia of Healing Foods*. New York: Atria Books, 2005.

Neal, Bill. *Gardener's Latin: A Lexicon*. Chapel Hill, NC: Algonquin Books of Chapel Hill, 1992.

Peter, K. V. *Handbook of Herbs and Spices*, vol. 2, 2nd ed. Philadelphia: Woodhead Publishing, 2004.

Phaneuf, Holly. *Herbs Demystified: A Scientist Explains How the Most Common Herbal Remedies Really Work*. New York: Marlowe & Company, 2005.

Ravindran, P. N. *The Encyclopedia of Herbs and Spices*. Boston: CABI, 2017.

Saberi, Helen. *Tea: A Global History*. London: Reaktion Books, Ltd., 2010.

Seymour, Miranda. *A Brief History of Thyme and Other Herbs*. New York: Grove Press, 2002.

Shah, Gagan, Richa Shri, Vivek Panchal, Narender Sharma, Bharpur Singh, and A. S. Mann. "Scientific basis for the therapeutic use of *Cymbopogon citratus*, stapf (Lemon grass)." *Journal of Advanced Pharmaceutical Technology & Research*, 2011 vol. 2(1), 3–8. http://www.japtr.org/text.asp?201½/⅓/79796 accessed 1/14/19.

Shealy, C. Norman. *The Healing Remedies Sourcebook: Over 1000 Natural Remedies to Prevent and Cure Common Ailments*. New York: HarperCollins Publishers, 2012.

Skidmore-Roth, Linda. *Mosby's Handbook of Herbs & Natural Supplements*, 4th ed. St. Louis, MO: Mosby Elsevier, 2010.

Staub, Jack. *75 Exceptional Herbs for Your Garden*. Layton, UT: Gibbs Smith, 2008.

Steel, Susannah, ed. *Home Herbal: Cook, Brew, and Blend Your Own Herbs*. New York: Dorling Kindersley Publishing, Inc., 2011.

Stein, Diane. *Healing Herbs A to Z: A Handy Reference to Healing Plants*. Berkeley, CA: Crossing Press, 2009.

Thacker, Holly L. *Women's Health: Your Body, Your Hormones, Your Choices: A Cleveland Clinic Guide*. Cleveland, OH: Cleveland Clinic Press, 2007.

Van Wyk, Ben-Erik, and Michael Wink. *Medicinal Plants of the World: An Illustrated Scientific Guide to Important Medicinal Plants and Their Uses*. Portland, OR: Timber Press, Inc., 2004.

index

To Write the Author

If you wish to contact the author or would like more information about this book, please write to the author in care of Llewellyn Worldwide, and we will forward your request. Both the author and publisher appreciate hearing from you and learning of your enjoyment of this book and how it has helped you. Llewellyn Worldwide cannot guarantee that every letter written to the author can be answered, but all will be forwarded. Please write to:

Sandra Kynes
℅ Llewellyn Worldwide
2143 Wooddale Drive
Woodbury, MN 55125.2989

Please enclose a self-addressed stamped envelope for reply, or $1.00 to cover costs. If outside the U.S.A., enclose an international postal reply coupon.

Many of Llewellyn's authors have websites with additional information and resources. For more information, please visit our website at http://www.llewellyn.com.